NATIONAL STRATEGY FOR THE COVID-19 RESPONSE AND PANDEMIC PREPAREDNESS

JANUARY 2021

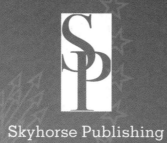

Skyhorse Publishing

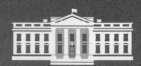

10 9 8 7 6 5 4 3 2 1

Library of Congress Cataloging-in-Publication Data is available on file.

ISBN: 978-1-5107-6760-7
eISBN: 978-1-5107-6761-4

Cover design by the United States Federal Government

Printed in the United States of America

TABLE OF CONTENTS

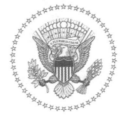

Letter from the President of the United States

My fellow Americans,

As I swore an oath to God and country to serve as your president, I offered a prayer for the 400,000 Americans and counting who have lost their lives this past year from the once-in-a-century pandemic in our midst. They were mothers and fathers, husbands and wives, sons and daughters, friends, neighbors, and colleagues who leave behind grieving loved ones and a nation on edge.

For the past year, we could not turn to the federal government for a national plan to answer prayers with action — until today. In the following pages, you will find my Administration's national strategy to beat the COVID-19 pandemic. It is a comprehensive plan that starts with restoring public trust and mounting an aggressive, safe, and effective vaccination campaign. It continues with the steps we know that stop the spread liked expanded masking, testing, and social distancing. It's a plan where the federal government works with states, cities, Tribal communities, and private industry to increase supply and administer testing and the vaccines that will help reopen schools and businesses safely. Equity will also be central to our strategy so that the communities and people being disproportionately infected and killed by the pandemic receive the care they need and deserve.

Our national strategy will be driven by scientists and public health experts who will regularly speak directly to you, free from political interference as they make decisions strictly on science and public health alone.

Above all, Vice President Harris and I, and our entire Administration, will always be honest and transparent with you about both the good news and the bad. The honest truth is we are still in a dark winter of this pandemic. It will get worse before it gets better. Progress will take time to measure as people getting infected today don't show up in case counts for weeks, and those who perish from the disease die weeks after exposure. Even as we make progress, we will face setbacks. But I know we can do it, and that a true national strategy will take all of us working together. It will take Congress providing the necessary funding. Families and neighbors will need to continue looking out for one another. We will need health care providers, businesses, civic, religious and civil rights organizations, and unions all rallying together in common purpose and with urgency, purpose, and resolve. We will need to reassert America's leadership in the world in the fight against this and future public health threats.

There are moments in history when more is asked of us as Americans. We are in that moment now and history will measure whether we were up to a task. Beating this pandemic will be one of the most difficult operational challenges we have ever faced as a nation. I believe we are ready, as fellow Americans and as the United States of America.

May God bless the lost souls of this pandemic, and all of you on the frontlines who define the best of who we are as Americans.

Sincerely,

Joe Biden

President Joe Biden

Executive Summary

☆ ☆ ☆ ☆ ☆ ☆

We can and will beat COVID-19. America deserves a response to the COVID-19 pandemic that is driven by science, data, and public health — not politics. Through the release of the National Strategy for the COVID-19 Response and Pandemic Preparedness, the United States is initiating a coordinated pandemic response that not only improves the effectiveness of our fight against COVID-19, but also helps restore trust, accountability and a sense of common purpose in our response to the pandemic.

On January 9, 2020, the World Health Organization announced that there were 59 cases of coronavirus-related pneumonia. Just one year later, the United States has experienced over 24 million confirmed COVID-19 cases and over 400,000 COVID-19 deaths. America has just 4% of the world's population, but 25% of the world's COVID-19 cases and 20% of all COVID-19 deaths. And our nation continues to experience the darkest days of the pandemic, with record numbers of cases, hospitalizations and deaths. Over 77,000 Americans lost their lives to COVID-19 in December, and across our nation businesses are closing, hospitals are full, and families are saying goodbye to their loved ones remotely.

The National Strategy provides a roadmap to guide America out of the worst public health crisis in a century. It outlines an actionable plan across the federal government to address the COVID-19 pandemic, including twelve initial executive actions issued by President Biden on his first two days in office:

The National Strategy is organized around seven goals:

1. **Restore trust with the American people.**
2. **Mount a safe, effective, and comprehensive vaccination campaign.**
3. **Mitigate spread through expanding masking, testing, data, treatments, health care workforce, and clear public health standards.**
4. **Immediately expand emergency relief and exercise the Defense Production Act.**
5. **Safely reopen schools, businesses, and travel while protecting workers.**

6. Protect those most at risk and advance equity, including across racial, ethnic and rural/urban lines.

7. Restore U.S. leadership globally and build better preparedness for future threats.

To execute on the National Strategy, the White House will establish a COVID-19 Response Office responsible for coordinating the pandemic response across all federal departments and agencies. Through implementation of the National Strategy, the United States will make immediate progress on the seven goals. To monitor outcomes, the National Strategy includes the creation of publicly accessible performance dashboards, establishing a data-driven, evidence-based approach to evaluating America's progress in the fight against COVID-19.

The federal government cannot solve this crisis alone. Full implementation of the National Strategy for COVID-19 will require sustained, coordinated, and complementary efforts of the American people, as well as groups across the country, including State, local, territorial, and Tribal governments; health care providers; businesses; manufacturers critical to the supply chain, communities of color, and unions. It will also require a global effort to contain the virus and advance health security.

America has always risen to the challenge we face and we will do so now. In collaboration with the people of this country, the United States government will lead an effective COVID-19 response that turns this crisis into a crucible, from which our nation will forge a stronger, better, and more equitable future.

GOAL 1

Restore trust with the American people.

The federal government should be the source of truth for the public to get clear, accessible, and scientifically accurate information about COVID-19. To rebuild the trust of the American people, the National Strategy will signal clear public leadership and a commitment to a robust whole-of-government response that puts science first. The federal government will be transparent with the American people, maintaining an open line of communication with the public and all stakeholders. To continue to restore trust, the United States will:

Establish a national COVID-19 response structure where decision-making is driven by science and equity. The Biden-Harris Administration has developed a unified plan to rebuild expert leadership across the government and regain the trust of the American public. As part of the strategy, on his first day in office, President Biden issued Executive Order *Organizing and Mobilizing the U.S. Government to Provide a Unified And Effective Response to Combat COVID-19 and to Provide United States Leadership on Global Health and Security* establishing a White House COVID-19 national response structure to coordinate across the U.S. Government and restoring the White House Directorate on Global Health Security and Biodefense established by the Obama-Biden Administration. The COVID-19 Response office will establish clear lines of communications with all governors, state public health officials and immunization managers, and local leaders.

Conduct regular expert-led, science-based public briefings. The federal government will conduct regular, expert-led, science-based public briefings and release regular reports on the state of the pandemic. Experts and scientists at the U.S. Centers for Disease Control and Prevention (CDC) will also develop clear, evidence-based, metric-driven public health guidance and effectively and frequently communicate and distribute guidance and updates to the American people.

Publicly share data around key response indicators. Metrics and metric-driven public health guidance will be essential to controlling the pandemic. President Biden issued Executive Order *Ensuring a Data-Driven Response to COVID-19 and Future High Consequence Public Health Threats* directing steps to enhance federal agencies' collection, production sharing, and analysis of, and collaboration with respect to, data to support an equitable COVID-19 response and recovery. As further detailed in National Strategy Goals Two, Three, and Six, the federal government will track a range of performance measures and data including cases, testing, vaccinations, and hospital admissions, and will make real-time information readily available to the public and to policymakers at the federal, state, and local level. The CDC will also maintain a public dashboard tracking COVID-19 cases at the county level, so that Americans can gauge the level of transmission in their own communities to make their own informed choices.

Engage the American people. The federal government cannot solve this crisis alone. It will take regular engagement with the public, state and local leaders, the private sector, unions, community volunteers, and health care providers to guide policy and implementation. The Administration will prioritize outreach to state and local governments, the public and private sectors, vulnerable communities, students, workers, and community leaders, using input from these stakeholders to drive the government's COVID-19 response.

Lead science-first public health campaigns. The Administration will lead world-class public education campaigns — covering topics like masking, testing, vaccinations and vaccine hesitancy — designed with diversity and inclusivity in mind, including communications in multiple languages, to maximize reach and effectiveness. The campaigns will be coordinated, across national, state, and local levels, and engage with the private and public sector. They will be anchored by science and fact-based public health guidance. The Administration will work to counter misinformation and disinformation by ensuring that Americans are obtaining science-based information.

GOAL 2

Mount a safe, effective, comprehensive vaccination campaign.

The United States will spare no effort to ensure Americans can get vaccinated quickly, effectively, and equitably. The federal government will execute an aggressive vaccination strategy, focusing on the immediate actions necessary to convert vaccines into vaccinations, including improving allocation, distribution, administration, and tracking. Central to this effort will be additional support and funding for state, local, Tribal, and territorial governments — and improved line of sight into supply — to ensure that they are best prepared to mount local vaccination programs. At the same time, the federal government will mount an unprecedented public campaign that builds trust around vaccination and communicates the importance of maintaining public health measures such as masking, physical distancing, testing, and contact tracing even as people receive safe and effective vaccinations. To mount a safe, effective, comprehensive vaccination campaign, the United States will:

Ensure the availability of safe, effective vaccines for the American public. The national vaccination effort will be one of the greatest operational challenges America has ever faced. To ensure all Americans can be vaccinated quickly, the President has developed a plan for expanding vaccine manufacturing and purchasing COVID-19 vaccine doses for the U.S. population by fully leveraging contract authorities, including the Defense Production Act; deploying onsite support to monitor contract manufacturing operations; and purchasing additional FDA-authorized vaccines to deliver as quickly as possible. The effort includes prioritizing supplies that could cause bottlenecks, including glass vials, stoppers, syringes, needles, and the "fill and finish" capacity to package vaccine into vials.

Accelerate getting shots into arms and get vaccines to the communities that need them most. The success of the national vaccination effort will depend on reaching communities across the United States. To achieve this, the federal government will take a series of steps to simplify and strengthen the allocation and distribution process. In order to expand the supply available to states, the Administration will end the policy of holding back significant levels of doses, instead holding back a small reserve and monitoring supply to ensure that everyone receives the full regimen as recommended by the FDA. The United States will accelerate the pace of vaccinations by encouraging states and localities to move through the priority groups more quickly — expanding access to frontline essential workers and individuals over the age of 65, while staying laser-focused on working to ensure that the highest-risk members of the public, including those in congregate facilities, can access the vaccine where and when they need it. The Administration will also improve the allocation process by providing states and localities with clear, consistent projections to inform their planning. Through it all, the United States will work to ensure that the vaccine is distributed quickly, effectively and equitably, with a focus on making sure that high-risk and hard-to-reach communities are not left behind.

Create as many venues as needed for people to be vaccinated. The federal government — in partnership with state and local governments — will create as many venues for vaccination as needed in communities and settings that people trust. This includes, but is not limited to federally run community vaccination centers, in places like stadiums and conference centers, federally-supported state and locally operated vaccination sites in all 50 states and 14 territories, pharmacies and retail stores, federal facilities like Veterans Affairs hospitals, community health centers, rural health clinics, critical access hospitals, physician offices, health systems, urgent care centers, and mobile and on-site occupational clinics.

Focus on hard-to-reach and high-risk populations. As the United States accelerates the pace of vaccinations nationwide, we remain focused on building programs to meet the needs of hard-to-reach and high-risk populations, and meeting communities where they are to make vaccinations as accessible and equitable as possible. The federal government will deploy targeted strategies to meet the needs of individuals at increased risk and others who need to take extra precautions, according to the CDC, as well as the communities hardest hit by this pandemic. Local public health officials will play a critical role.

Fairly compensate providers, and states and local governments for the cost of administering vaccinations. Fairly compensating providers, and state and local governments for the costs of vaccine administration will be critical to expanding vaccination participation. President Biden will work with Congress to expand the Federal Medicaid Assistance Percentage (FMAP) to 100 percent for vaccinations of Medicaid enrollees—with the goal of alleviating state costs for administration of these vaccines and supporting states in their work to meet the needs of their communities. The Department of Health and Human Services will ask the Centers for Medicare & Medicaid Services to consider whether current payment rates for vaccine administration are appropriate or whether a higher rate may more accurately compensate providers. The federal government will fund vaccine supply and will greatly expand funding for vaccine administration by allowing state and local governments to reimburse vaccination administration expenses through the FEMA Disaster Relief Fund and by ensuring that workforce and equipment expenses for state and local-run sites are also eligible.

Drive equity throughout the vaccination campaign and broader pandemic response. The federal government will drive equity in vaccinations by using demographic data to identify communities hit hardest by the virus and supporting them, ensuring no out-of-pocket costs for vaccinations, and making sure vaccines reach those communities. Working with state, local, and community-based organizations and trusted health care providers, like community health centers, will be central to this effort.

Launch a national vaccinations public education campaign. The United States will build public trust through an unprecedented vaccination public health campaign at the federal, State, Tribal, territorial, local and community level. The public education campaign will support vaccination programs, address vaccine hesitancy, help simplify the vaccination process for Americans, and educate the public on effective prevention measures. The campaign will be tailored to meet the needs of diverse communities, get information to trusted, local messengers, and outline efforts to deliver a safe and effective vaccine as part of a national strategy for beating COVID-19.

Bolster data systems and transparency for vaccinations. The operational complexity of vaccinating the public will make robust data and its use in decision-making related to vaccinations more important than ever. The federal government, with CDC, will track distribution and vaccination progress, working hand-in-hand with states and localities to support their efforts. The Administration will build on and strengthen the federal government's approach to data collection related to vaccination efforts, removing impediments and developing communication and technical assistance plans for jurisdictions and providers. The Administration, through HHS and other federal partners, will rely on data to drive decision-making and the national vaccinations program.

Monitor vaccine safety and efficacy. The Administration will ensure that scientists are in charge of all decisions related to vaccine safety and efficacy. The FDA will also continue to honor its commitment to make relevant data on vaccine safety and efficacy publicly available and to provide opportunities for public, non-governmental expert input. Through expanded and existing systems, the CDC and FDA will ensure ongoing, real-time safety monitoring. Through it all, the Administration will communicate clearly with the American public to continue to build trust around the vaccine and its benefits for individuals, their families and communities.

Surge the health care workforce to support the vaccination effort. A diverse, community-based health care workforce is essential to an effective vaccination program. The United States will address workforce needs by taking steps to allow qualified professionals to administer vaccines and encourage states to leverage their flexibility fully to surge their workforce, including by expanding scope of practice laws and waiving licensing requirements as appropriate.

GOAL 3

Mitigate spread through expanding masking, testing, treatment, data, workforce, and clear public health standards.

A comprehensive national public health effort to control the virus — even after the vaccination program ramps up — will be critical to saving lives and restoring economic activity. The federal government will partner with state, local, Tribal, and territorial leaders to implement a cohesive strategy to significantly reduce the spread of COVID-19 and release clear public health guidance to the public about what to do and when, including implementing mask mandates; expanding testing; strengthening the public health workforce; modernizing data collection and reporting capabilities for COVID-19 and future epidemics; and providing equitable access to treatment and clinical care. To mitigate the spread of COVID-19 through clear public health standards, the United States will:

Implement masking nationwide by working with governors, mayors, and the American people. The President has asked the American people to do what they do best: step up in a time of crisis and wear masks. He has issued Executive Order *Protecting the Federal Workforce and Requiring Mask-Wearing* which directs compliance with CDC guidance on masking and physical distancing in federal buildings, on federal lands, and by federal employees and contractors. Additionally, the President issued Executive Order *Promoting COVID-19 Safety in Domestic and International Travel* which directs applicable agencies to take immediate action to require mask-wearing on many airplanes, trains, and certain other forms of public transportation in the United States. He has called on governors, public health officials, mayors, business leaders, and others to implement masking, physical distancing, and other CDC public measures to control COVID-19.

Scale and expand testing. To control the COVID-19 pandemic and safely reopen schools and businesses, America must have wide-spread testing. A national testing strategy is a cornerstone to reducing the spread of COVID-19 and controlling outbreaks, and clear federal guidance and a unified national approach to implementation are essential. The President issued Executive Order *Establishing the National Pandemic Testing Board and Ensuring a Sustainable Public Health Workforce for COVID-19 and Other Biological Threats* which establishes the COVID-19 Pandemic Testing Board to oversee implementation of a clear, unified approach to testing. The federal government will expand the rapid testing supply and double test supplies and increase testing capacity. The Administration will also increase onshore test manufacturing, fill testing supply shortfalls, enhance laboratory capacity to conduct testing over the short- and long-term, and expand surveillance for hotspots and variants.

Effectively distribute tests and expand access to testing. The federal government will support school screening testing programs to help schools reopen. The Administration will also stand up a dedicated CDC Testing Support Team, fund rapid test acquisition and distribution for priority populations, work to spur development and manufacturing of at-home tests and work to ensure that tests are widely available. Through Executive Order *Establishing the National Pandemic Testing Board and Ensuring a Sustainable Public Health Workforce for COVID-19 and Other Biological Threats* the President directs agencies to facilitate testing free of charge for those who lack health insurance and to clarify insurers' obligation to cover testing. The federal government will also provide testing protocols to inform the use of testing in congregate settings, schools, and other critical areas and among asymptomatic individuals. Further, technical assistance will support more widespread adoption of testing to improve timely diagnosis and public confidence in the safety of settings like schools.

Prioritize therapeutics and establish a comprehensive, integrated COVID-19 treatment discovery and development program. Effective treatments for COVID-19 are critical to saving lives. The federal government will establish a comprehensive, integrated, and coordinated preclinical drug discovery and development program, with diverse clinical trials, to allow therapeutics to be evaluated and developed rapidly in response to COVID-19 and other pandemic threats. This includes promoting the immediate and rapid development of therapeutics that respond to COVID-19 by developing new antivirals directed against the coronavirus family, accelerating research and support for clinical trials for therapeutics in response to COVID-19 with a focus on those that can be readily scaled and administered, and developing broad-spectrum antivirals to prevent future viral pandemics. President Biden issued Executive Order *Improving and Expanding Access to Care and Treatment for COVID-19* which also outlines steps to bolster clinical care capacity, provide assistance to long-term care facilities and intermediate care facilities for people with disabilities, increase health care workforce capacity, expand access to programs designed to meet long-term health needs of patients recovering from COVID-19, and support access to safe and effective COVID-19 therapies for those without coverage.

Develop actionable, evidence-based public health guidance. CDC will develop and update public health guidance on containment and mitigation that provides metrics for measuring and monitoring the incidence and prevalence of COVID-19 in health care facilities, schools, workplaces, and the general public, including metric-driven reopening guidance that the federal government communicates widely. Informed by up-to-date national and state data, the CDC will provide and update guidance on key issues such as physical distancing protocols, testing, contact tracing, reopening schools and businesses, and masking. The CDC also will provide focused guidance for older Americans and others at higher risk, including people with disabilities.

Expand the U.S. public health workforce and increase clinical care capacity for COVID-19. In addition to supporting the surge in health care workers for vaccination efforts detailed in Goal Two, the federal government will also build and support an effective public health workforce to fight COVID-19 and the next public health threat. As part of the President's commitment to provide 100,000 COVID-19 contact tracers, community health workers, and public health nurses, the Administration will establish a U.S. Public Health Jobs Corps, provide support for community health workers, and mobilize Americans to support communities most at-risk. The United States will also provide technical support for testing, contact tracing, and other urgent public health workforce needs to better prepare for public health crises.

Improve data to guide the response to COVID-19. Federal agencies will make increased use of data to guide the public health response against COVID-19. To that end, Agencies will collect, aggregate, share, and analyze non-personally identifiable data, and take steps to make it publicly available and in a machine-readable form to enhance COVID-19 response efforts. And the federal government will facilitate evidence-based decision-making through focused data-based projects. These efforts will require collaboration with state, local, Tribal, and territorial governments to aggregate and analyze data for critical decisions to track access to vaccines and testing, reopen schools and businesses, address disparities in COVID-19 infections and health outcomes, and enhance critical monitoring capacity where needed. In addition, critical response activities such as workforce mobilization and vaccination appointment scheduling may require new technology solutions. The federal government will provide technical support to ensure that these systems meet mission critical requirements to support a robust response.

GOAL 4

Immediately expand emergency relief and exercise the Defense Production Act.

It's past time to fix America's COVID-response supply shortage problems for good. The United States will immediately address urgent supply gaps, which will require monitoring and strengthening supply chains, while also steering the distribution of supplies to areas with the greatest need. As new vaccines, testing protocols, and treatments are developed, they will also need to be manufactured in sufficient supply. To respond to this unprecedented operational challenge, the President is immediately expanding emergency relief by giving state and local governments the support they need. To make vaccines, tests, Personal Protective Equipment (PPE), and other critical supplies available for the duration of the pandemic, the President has directed the use of all available legal authorities, including the Defense Production Act (DPA), instructing departments and agencies to expand the availability of critical supplies, to increase stockpiles so that PPE is available to be used in the recommended safe manner, and to start to fill all supply shortfalls immediately. To expand emergency relief and strengthen the supply chain, the government will:

Increase emergency funding to states and bolster the Federal Emergency Management Agency (FEMA) response. The President has issued a Presidential Memorandum entitled *Extend Federal Support to Governors' Use of National Guard to Respond to COVID-19 and to Increase Reimbursement and other Assistance Provided to States*, directing FEMA to fully reimburse states for the cost of National Guard personnel and emergency supplies, including emergency supplies like PPE for schools and child care providers.

Fill supply shortfalls by invoking the Defense Production Act (DPA). The United States is taking immediate action to fill supply shortfalls for vaccination supplies, testing supplies, and PPE. The President issued Executive Order *A Sustainable Public Health Supply Chain* which directs agencies to fill supply shortfalls using all available legal authorities, including the DPA, and the United States has identified twelve immediate supply shortfalls that will be critical to the pandemic response, including shortages in the dead-space needle syringes available to administer the vaccine. The President has directed relevant agencies to exercise all appropriate authorities, including the DPA, to accelerate manufacturing, delivery, and administration to meet shortfalls in these twelve categories of critical supplies, including taking action to increase the availability of supplies like N95 masks, isolation gowns, nitrile gloves, polymerase chain reaction (PCR) sample collection swabs, test reagents, pipette tips, laboratory analysis machines for PCR tests, high-absorbency foam swabs, nitrocellulose material for rapid antigen tests, rapid test kits, low dead-space needles and syringes, and all the necessary equipment and material to accelerate the manufacture, delivery, and administration of COVID-19 vaccine.

Identify and solve urgent COVID-19 related supply gaps and strengthen the supply chain. The *A Sustainable Public Health Supply Chain* executive order also directs federal agencies to fill supply shortfalls using all available legal authorities. The federal government will focus on the near-term goal of building a stable, secure, and resilient supply chain with increased domestic manufacturing in four key critical sectors:

- Antigen and molecular-based testing;
- PPE and durable medical equipment;
- Vaccine development and manufacturing; and
- Therapeutics and key drugs.

The federal government will immediately focus on procuring supplies that will be critical to control the spread of COVID-19 by initiating contracts, entering into purchase commitments, making investments to produce supplies and expanding manufacturing capacity.

Secure the pandemic supply chain and create a manufacturing base in the United States. To respond more effectively to this crisis, and ensure that the United States is able to respond more quickly and efficiently to the next pandemic, we need a resilient, domestic public health industrial base. The U.S. Government will not only secure supplies for fighting the COVID-19 pandemic, but also build toward a future, flexible supply chain and expand an American manufacturing capability where the United States is not dependent on other countries in a crisis. To this end, *A Sustainable Public Health Supply Chain* directs the development of a new Pandemic Supply Chain Resilience Strategy.

Improve distribution and expand availability of critical materials. After conducting a review of existing COVID-19 and related pandemic supply chain distribution plans and working in consultation with state and regional compacts, the United States will coordinate distribution plans, prioritizing areas of highest-risk and highest need, and set up a structure to improve the distribution of critical materials. To work toward expanding the affordability and accessibility of supplies, *A Sustainable Public Health Supply Chain* directs the Department of Defense (DOD), HHS, and Department of Homeland Security (DHS) to develop recommendations to address the pricing of COVID-19 supplies. The federal government will also reduce the opacity of the market for critical supplies and supply chains by clearly and rapidly communicating with states, health care providers, and manufacturers about federal interventions.

GOAL 5

Safely reopen schools, businesses, and travel, while protecting workers.

Reopening schools, businesses, travel, and our economy will require major, unified federal investments in rapid testing, an expanded rapid response public health workforce, clear guidance and protections, and support for people to stay home when they are infected to stop the spread of COVID-19. At the same time that the United States takes immediate steps to achieve an overall decrease in COVID-19 spread, it will also support the safe operation of schools, businesses, and travel. To protect workers and safely reopen, schools, businesses, and travel, the United States will:

Implement a national strategy to support safely reopening schools. The United States is committed to ensuring that students and educators are able to resume safe, in-person learning as quickly as possible, with the goal of getting a majority of K-8 schools safely open in 100 days. The President issued Executive Order *Supporting the Reopening and Continuing Operation of Schools and Early Childhood Education Providers* which directs a national strategy for safely reopening schools, including requiring the Departments of Education and HHS to provide guidance on safe reopening and operating, and to develop a Safer Schools and Campuses Best Practices Clearinghouse to share lessons learned and best practices from across the country. Presidential Memorandum *Extend Federal Support to Governors' Use of National Guard to Respond to COVID-19 and to Increase Reimbursement and other Assistance Provided to States* restores full reimbursement for eligible costs necessary to support safe school reopening through the FEMA Disaster Relief Fund and the President has called on Congress to provide at least $130 billion in dedicated funding to schools, $350 billion in flexible state and local relief funds that will help districts avoid lay-offs and close budget gaps, and additional resources so that schools can safely reopen, including funds to implement screening testing. The Administration will release a handbook that helps schools and local leaders implement the precautions and strategies necessary for safe reopening. It will also work with states and local school districts to support screening testing in schools, including working with states to ensure an adequate supply of test kits.

Support safe operations at child care centers and at-home providers. With enrollments down and costs up due to COVID-19 precautions, child care providers are struggling to stay afloat while providing vital services to their communities. Due to increased costs and lower enrollment, a recent survey of child care providers showed that most child care providers expect that they will close within a few months without relief, or are uncertain how long they can stay open.[1] If not addressed, child care providers will close and millions of parents will be left to make devastating choices between caring for their children and working to put food on the table. President Biden has called on Congress to provide $25 billion in emergency stabilization to support hard-hit child care providers through the pandemic. These funds would help providers pay rent, utilities, and payroll, as well as cover pandemic-related costs like personal protective equipment, ventilation supplies, smaller group sizes, and alterations to physical spaces that improve safety. The President has also called on Congress to provide $15 billion to help families struggling to afford child care.

---

[1] https://www.naeyc.org/sites/default/files/globally-shared/downloads/PDFs/our-work/public-policy-advocacy/naeyc_policy_crisis_coronavirus_december_survey_data.pdf

Support equitable reopening and operation in higher education. College enrollment for high school graduates was down more than 20% in 2020 compared to 2019, and students from low-income families are nearly twice as likely to report canceling their plans to attend college. Reopening and keeping colleges open is critical to ensuring that all Americans have a shot at a college credential — but it must be done safely, to protect the health of students, faculty, staff, and the broader community. To support colleges through the pandemic, President Biden has requested that Congress provide an additional $35 billion in emergency stabilization funds for higher education.

Protect workers and issue stronger worker safety guidance. It is critical that the federal government protect the health and safety of America's workers and take swift action to prevent workers from contracting COVID-19 in the workplace. The President issued Executive Order *Protecting Worker Health and Safety* which directs the Occupational Safety and Health Administration (OSHA) to issue updated guidance on COVID-19 worker protections. It also directs OSHA and the Mine Safety and Health Administration (MSHA) to consider whether emergency temporary standards, including with respect to mask-wearing, are necessary. President Biden is taking steps to cover workers not typically covered by OSHA or MSHA by directing agencies like the Department of Transportation to keep workers safe. He has also called on Congress to extend and expand emergency paid leave; to allow OSHA to issue standards covering a broad set of workers, like many public workers on the frontlines; to provide additional funding for worker health and safety enforcement, and to provide grant funding for organizations to help keep vulnerable workers healthy and safe from COVID-19.

Provide guidance and support to safely open businesses. To maintain safe operations during the pandemic, businesses need to know how to change their practices to protect employees and customers. As the conditions of the pandemic continue to evolve and more Americans get vaccinated, the business community needs clear information from the federal government on what to expect and how to adapt their operations. Many businesses affected by the pandemic–particularly the smallest ones–need additional support to adjust their physical spaces and purchase PPE and supplies. The United States will immediately work to prioritize funds under the recent COVID relief package to the companies hardest hit by COVID-19 and in compliance with public health restrictions, ensuring that small businesses have the funds they need to operate safely. Further, the Small Business Administration will work with the Department of Labor to disseminate updated OSHA guidance on worker safety and support businesses in implementing the updated guidance.

Promote Safe Travel. Ensuring that people can safely travel will be critical for families and to jumpstarting the economy, which is why the President issued an executive order that requires mask-wearing on certain public modes of transportation and at ports of entry to the United States. For international air travel, Executive Order *Promoting COVID-19 Safety in Domestic and International Travel* requires a recent negative COVID-19 test result prior to departure and quarantine on arrival, consistent with CDC guidelines. The Executive Order also directs agencies to develop options for expanding public health measures for domestic travel and cross-border land and sea travel and calls for incentives to support and encourage compliance with CDC guidelines on public transportation.

GOAL 6

Protect those most at risk and advance equity, including across racial, ethnic and rural/urban lines.

The COVID-19 pandemic has exposed and exacerbated severe and pervasive health inequities among communities defined by race, ethnicity, geography, disability, sexual orientation, gender identity, and other factors. Addressing this pandemic's devastating toll is both a moral imperative and pragmatic policy. The federal government will address disparities in rates of infection, illness and death. Each of the goals of this National Strategy include comprehensive actions that will address these disparities and advance equity. In addition, the United States will:

Establish the COVID-19 Health Equity Task Force. The President issued Executive Order *Ensuring an Equitable Pandemic Response and Recovery* which establishes a high-level task force to address COVID-19 related health and social inequities and help coordinate an equitable pandemic response and recovery. The Task Force will convene national experts on health equity and provide recommendations on how to mitigate COVID-19 health inequities.

Increase data collection and reporting for high risk groups. The fragmented and limited availability of data by race, ethnicity, geography, disability and other demographic variables delays recognition of risk and a targeted response. President Biden issued the Executive Order *Ensuring a Data-Driven Response to COVID-19 and Future High-Consequence Public Health Threats* directing federal agencies to expand their data infrastructure to increase collection and reporting of health data for high risk populations, while reaffirming data privacy. Using these data, the federal government will identify high-risk communities, track resource distribution and evaluate the effectiveness of the response. Finally, HHS will optimize data collection from public and private entities to increase the availability of data by race, ethnicity, geography, disability, and other demographic variables, as feasible.

Ensure equitable access to critical COVID-19 PPE, tests, therapies and vaccines. The continued surge of COVID-19 highlights the critical importance of meaningful access to PPE, tests, therapies, and vaccines to prevent spread and reduce illness and death in high-risk populations and settings. The federal government will center equity in its COVID-19 response, providing PPE, tests, vaccines, therapeutics and other resources in a fair and transparent way. A targeted, stakeholder- and data-informed vaccination communication campaign will be launched to encourage vaccination in all communities. Additionally, the CDC will work with states and localities to update their pandemic plans. Finally, through prioritizing diverse and inclusive representation in clinical research and strengthening enforcement of anti-discrimination requirements, the federal government will increase access to effective COVID-19 care and treatment.

Expand access to high quality health care. The federal government will work to expand affordable coverage to increase access to care during this pandemic, and the Task Force will provide recommendations to align federal incentives with improved clinical outcomes. Specific actions include efforts to increase funding for community health centers, provide greater assistance to safety net institutions, strengthen home- and community-based services, expand mental health care, and support care and research on the effects of long COVID.

Expand the clinical and public health workforce, including community-based workers. In order to assure equitable PPE distribution, testing, contact tracing, social support for quarantine and isolation and vaccination, there must be sufficient workforce to serve the communities in greatest need. The federal government will augment the health workforce, including with community based workers, as outlined in Goal Three above, to help fill this critical gap. The federal government will create a United States Public Health Workforce Program of new community based workers to assist with testing, tracing and vaccination. Additionally, it will deploy federal workers to assist with the COVID-19 response in under-resourced areas.

Strengthen the social service safety net to address unmet basic needs. With millions of families already struggling pre-pandemic to meet basic needs, including food, housing and transportation, COVID-19 has exacerbated these challenges. These challenges contribute to difficulties by many to adhere to public health guidance regarding social distancing and quarantine/isolation. This Administration is committed to addressing these needs in multiple ways, including providing paid sick leave, child care support, and rental assistance, with requested Congressional appropriations. Additionally, it will undertake agency actions to designate COVID-19 health equity leads and extend eligibility and enrollment flexibilities for select programs during the pandemic, as well work with community-based, multi-sector organizations to align health and social interventions.

Support communities most at-risk for COVID-19. The federal government is committed to supporting populations that are most vulnerable to COVID-19. Whether residing in congregate settings (such as prisons, nursing and group homes, and homeless shelters), serving as essential workers, living as a person with a disability, or bearing the burden of chronic medical conditions, these vulnerable populations are disproportionately composed of people of color. The CDC will develop and update clear public health guidance for such high-risk populations and settings to further minimize the risk of COVID infection, and work with states to update their pandemic plans to incorporate such guidance as necessary.

GOAL 7

Restore U.S. leadership globally and build better preparedness for future threats.

U.S. international engagement to combat COVID-19, promote health, and advance global health security is urgent to save lives, promote economic recovery, and develop resilience against future biological catastrophes. America's withdrawal from the world stage has impeded progress on a global COVID-19 response and left the U.S. more vulnerable to future pandemics. The Biden-Harris Administration will restore America's role in leading the world through global crises, advancing global health security and the Global Health Security Agenda, including by supporting the international pandemic response effort, providing humanitarian relief and global health assistance, and building resilience for future epidemics and pandemics. The President has issued a National Security Directive that directs steps to restore U.S. leadership globally and build better preparedness. In addition, the United States of America will:

Restore the U.S. relationship with the World Health Organization and seek to strengthen and reform it. The World Health Organization (WHO) is essential to coordinating the international response to COVID-19 and improving the health of all people. On his first day in office, the President sent letters informing the UN Secretary-General and the WHO Director General of his decision to cease the previous Administration's process of withdrawal from the WHO and meet its financial obligations. The United States is participating in the WHO Executive Board meeting this month, and will take actions to strengthen and reform the WHO.

Surge the international COVID-19 public health & humanitarian response. The United States will commit to multilateralism in the international COVID-19 public health and humanitarian response. The President will restore U.S. leadership on the global COVID-19 response and health security, laying out an active role for the United States in surging the health and humanitarian response to COVID-19, and supporting global vaccine distribution and research and development for treatments, tests, and vaccines. The United States will support the Access to COVID-19 Tools (ACT) Accelerator, join the COVID-19 Vaccines Global Access (COVAX) Facility, and seek to strengthen other existing multilateral initiatives, such as the Coalition for Epidemic Preparedness Innovations; Gavi, the Vaccine Alliance; and the Global Fund to Fight AIDS, Tuberculosis, and Malaria. The United States will also take steps to enhance humanitarian relief and support for the capacity of the most vulnerable communities to prevent, detect, respond to, mitigate, and recover from impacts of COVID-19, such as food insecurity and gender-based violence.

Restore U.S. leadership to the international COVID-19 response and advance global health security and diplomacy. The United States will promote sustainable global health and global health security, rebuild health security alliances, elevate U.S. efforts to support the Global Health Security Agenda, and revitalize U.S. leadership. The United States will advance global health security financing, promote efforts to harmonize crisis response and early warning for public health emergencies, and strengthen global pandemic supply chains. The United States will also work within the UN Security Council and with partners to strengthen multilateral public health and humanitarian cooperation on the COVID-19 response, global institutions to combat disease, and a global health security architecture to prevent, detect, and respond to future biological threats.

Build better biopreparedness and expand resilience for biological threats. The United States is committed to strengthening U.S. biopreparedness and capacity to counter COVID-19 and future biological threats. The President has immediately restored the White House National Security Council Directorate for Global Health Security and Biodefense, originally established by the Obama-Biden administration. He has reconstituted White House and Administration-wide infrastructure for monitoring and responding to emerging biological risks. And to improve the United States' preparedness, the Administration will work to secure funding and Congressional support to establish an integrated, National Center for Epidemic Forecasting and Outbreak Analytics to modernize global early warning and trigger systems to prevent, detect, and respond to biological threats. The United States will also review and seek to strengthen our pandemic supply chain, public health workforce, medical countermeasure development and distribution, bioeconomic investment and technology-related risks.

INTRODUCTION

On January 9, 2020, the World Health Organization announced that there were 59 cases of coronavirus-related pneumonia. Just one year later, the United States has experienced over 24 million confirmed COVID-19 cases and over 400,000 COVID-19 deaths. America has just 4% of the world's population, but 25% of the world's COVID-19 cases and 20% of all COVID-19 deaths. And the virus has devastated many families - and had an even more severe impact on some communities: communities of color, low-income neighborhoods and individuals living in congregate settings like nursing homes and prisons.

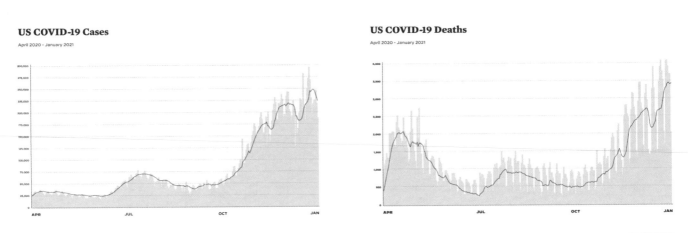

US COVID-19 Cases
April 2020 - January 2021

US COVID-19 Deaths
April 2020 - January 2021

Source: COVID Tracking Project

—— 7-day average

The United States has faced three waves of the pandemic: the first in the spring, centered in the Northeast, the second in the summer, centered in the south and southwest, and the current wave, where the virus has reached a point of uncontrolled spread across the country.

The current wave continues to be the longest, broadest and most severe, setting record after grim record and straining the health system across the country. While prior waves peaked in a little over five weeks, this current wave has lasted more than nine weeks, and our nation continues to experience the darkest days of the pandemic, with continuously rising case, death, and hospitalization counts. Across our nation schools and businesses are closed, hospitals are full and families are saying goodbye to their loved ones remotely.

COVID-19 Cases by Region over Time

April 2020 - January 2021

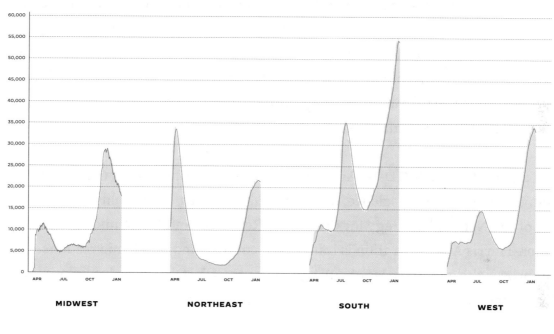

Source: COVID Tracking Project

— 7-day average

Since November 2020, there have been over 13 million cases, or more than all of the recorded cases from the start of the pandemic until that point. Hospitalizations have also hit record levels: every day since early December, there have been more than 100,000 Americans in the hospital due to the coronavirus. Hospitals and health care workers are strained nearly to the breaking point: hospitals and intensive care units are nearing or reaching capacity, some states are preparing for crisis standards of care, and at least one major county asked emergency medical workers to ration oxygen used to treat patients. Over 1,000 hospitals are reporting critical staffing shortages. Health care workers, who have been battling the pandemic for months on end, are exhausted, and the severe situation all across the country at once means that help cannot be brought in from other states.

Deaths have also reached unprecedented, tragic levels. There were more than 114,000 deaths in November and December, roughly the population of a mid-sized city, compared to 32,000 in the two months prior. We are on pace to have more new cases in January 2021 than in the first eight months of the pandemic, combined. National experts project as many as 48,000 to 81,000 more deaths in January alone.

Even as Americans endure a record surge, new mutations of the coronavirus pose the threat of even faster spread. Viruses regularly evolve, and at least four new variants of the coronavirus have been identified in recent weeks. The United States is not alone in this fight; the pandemic has impacted countries and people around the globe. The virus, including new variants in recent weeks, has laid bare the connections between our health and that of other countries. The variant originally found in the United Kingdom, known as B.1.1.7, has been identified in numerous states across the country and is found to be 30% - 70% more transmissible. In England and Ireland, the variant has spread explosively despite public health measures. It has now been identified in the United States as well. Other variants first detected in South Africa, Nigeria and Brazil are also potentially more transmissible and could impact the effectiveness of therapeutics and vaccines, or could make reinfection more likely.

We can and will beat COVID-19. America deserves a response to the COVID-19 pandemic that is driven by science, data, and public health — not politics. Through the release of the National Strategy for COVID-19 Response and Pandemic Preparedness, the Biden-Harris Administration is initiating a coordinated pandemic response that not only improves the effectiveness of our fight against COVID-19, but also helps restore trust, accountability and a sense of common purpose in our government.

The National Strategy provides a roadmap to guide America out of the worst public health crisis in a century. Including twelve initial executive actions issued by President Biden on his first two days in office, the National Strategy outlines an actionable plan across the federal government to combat COVID-19. The National Strategy will guide the activities of the Biden-Harris Administration in using all the powers of the federal government to address the COVID-19 pandemic.

THE NATIONAL STRATEGY IS ORGANIZED AROUND SEVEN GOALS:

- Restore trust with the American people.
- Mount a safe, effective, and comprehensive vaccination campaign.
- Mitigate spread through expanding masking, testing, treatments, data, health care workforce, and clear public health standards.
- Immediately expand emergency relief and exercise the Defense Production Act.
- Safely reopen schools, businesses, and travel while protecting workers.
- Protect those most at risk and advance equity, including across racial, ethnic and rural/urban lines.
- Restore U.S. leadership globally and build better preparedness for future threats.

If Americans come together, persevere, reinvest in proven public health strategies, and work with our partners around the globe, we can rise to the challenging moment and beat this virus. To execute on the National Strategy, the White House will establish a COVID-19 Response Office responsible for coordinating the pandemic response across all federal departments and agencies. Through implementation of the National Strategy, the United States will make immediate progress on the seven goals. To monitor outcomes, the National Strategy establishes a data-driven, evidence-based approach to evaluating America's progress in the fight against COVID-19.

The federal government cannot solve this crisis alone. Full implementation of the National Strategy for COVID-19 will require sustained, coordinated, and complementary efforts of the American people, as well as groups across the country, including State, local, territorial, and Tribal governments; health care providers; businesses; manufacturers critical to the supply chain; civic, religious and civil rights organizations, and unions. It will also require a global effort to contain the virus and advance health security.

America has always risen to the moment when confronted with difficult challenges, and we will do so now. In collaboration with the people of this country, the United States government will lead an effective COVID-19 response that gets us back to our lives and loved ones. As we've seen during this pandemic, we can't solve our problems as a divided nation. The only way we come through this is together as fellow Americans and as the United States of America.

Restore trust with the American people

KEY ACTIONS

— Establish a national COVID-19 response structure where decision-making is driven by science and equity.
— Conduct regular expert-led, science-based public briefings.
— Publicly share data around key response indicators.
— Engage the American people.
— Lead science-first public health campaigns

IMMEDIATE ACTIONS

The President has taken immediate action to implement goal one of the National Strategy by establishing a clear, organized, COVID-19 Response structure in the federal government.

— Executive Order: Organizing and Mobilizing the U.S. Government to Provide a Unified And Effective Response to Combat COVID-19 and to Provide United States Leadership on Global Health and Security (January 20, 2021).

EXECUTIVE ORDER ISSUED

President Biden issued Executive Order *Organizing and Mobilizing the U.S. Government to Provide a Unified And Effective Response to Combat COVID-19 and to Provide United States Leadership on Global Health and Security* establishing a White House COVID-19 national response structure to coordinate across the U.S. Government and restoring the White House Directorate on Global Health Security and Biodefense established by the Obama-Biden Administration.

The federal government should be the source of truth for the public to get clear, accessible, and scientifically accurate information about COVID-19. To rebuild the trust of the American people, the federal actions in the National Strategy signal clear public leadership and a commitment to a robust whole of government response that puts science first. The federal government will be transparent with the American people, maintaining an open line of communication with the public and all all stakeholders. To continue to restore trust, the United States will:

Establish a national COVID-19 response structure where decision-making is driven by science and equity. The Biden-Harris Administration has developed a unified plan to rebuild expert leadership across the government and regain the trust of an American public. As part of the strategy, on his first day in office, President Biden issued Executive Order *Organizing and Mobilizing the U.S. Government to Provide a Unified And Effective Response to Combat COVID-19 and to Provide United States Leadership on Global Health and Security* establishing a White House COVID-19 national response structure to coordinate across the U.S. Government and restoring the White House Directorate on Global Health Security and Biodefense established by the Obama-Biden Administration. The White House COVID-19 Response office will establish clear channels with all governors, state public health officials and immunization managers, and local leaders for proactive communications and rapid response.

● **Establish a COVID-19 National Response Structure.** The President signed Executive Order *Organizing and Mobilizing the U.S. Government to Provide a Unified And Effective Response to Combat COVID-19 and to Provide United States Leadership on Global Health and Security* establishing a White House-led national COVID-19 response structure to coordinate across the U.S. Government in responding to the COVID-19 pandemic. The duties of the office include coordinating a government-wide effort to produce, supply, and distribute personal protective equipment, vaccines, tests, and other supplies for the COVID-19 response; coordinating the timely, safe, and effective delivery of COVID-19 vaccines to the American public; coordinating the federal government's efforts to support the safe reopening and operation of schools, child care providers, and Head Start programs; and coordinating efforts to reduce disparities in response, care, and treatment of COVID-19. The Executive Order also restores the White House Directorate on Global Health Security and Biodefense established by the Obama-Biden Administration and restores White House infrastructure to monitor and rapidly respond to emerging domestic and global biological threats and pandemics.

● **Build clear channels of communication with state and local leaders.** The federal government will build clear channels of communication and engagement — including regular standing meetings — with governors, mayors, county executives, Tribal, territorial leaders, and state and local public health officials and immunization managers to execute on a unified federal COVID-19 response, accounting for state and local inventory, community needs, and supply and testing gaps. The national COVID-19 response structure will facilitate coordinated federal, State, local, Tribal, and territorial vaccination planning, masking and physical distancing planning; as well as surge testing and workforce planning to reopen schools and businesses. Clear channels between federal, state and local governments will also enable immediate, coordinated rapid response efforts.

● **Lead a coordinated, federal response that includes elevates the voices of public health experts.** The COVID-19 Response Team will lead a coordinated national response structure across all of the federal agencies of the U.S. Government that includes the voices of public health officials. The Administration will lead with science and scientists with a Centers for Disease Control and Prevention and National Institutes of Health that are free from political influence, a Surgeon General who is independent and speaks directly to the people, and an FDA whose decisions are based on science and science alone. These public-health experts, as well as the President, will communicate regularly with the public and drive a clear, unified, and consistent message that can be carried at the national, state, Tribal, and local levels and by the public and private sector.

Conduct regular expert-led, science-based public briefings. The federal government will conduct regular, expert-led, science-based public briefings and release regular reports on the state of the pandemic. Experts and scientists at the U.S. Centers for Disease Control and Prevention (CDC) will also develop clear, evidence-based, metric-driven public health guidance and effectively and frequently communicate and distribute that guidance and updates to the American people.

● **Conduct regular science-based, expert-led public briefings.** The federal government will provide regular briefings led by public health experts and officials. All COVID-19 briefings will be based on science, evidence, and public health.

● **Communicate clear, evidence-based public health guidance.** Experts and scientists at the CDC will develop, release, update or reissue public health guidance on COVID-19 containment, mitigation, as well as metrics for measuring and monitoring progress for health care facilities, schools, businesses, workplaces, and the general public. Clear public health guidance will be accessible and affirmatively communicated to all local and state leaders, as well as the general public.

● **Release a science-based, data-driven, regular report to the public.** The federal government will release a regular report, which will be authored by scientists and public health experts and include critical data on vaccinations, testing, supplies, contact tracing, and the public health workforce. Metrics and recommendations will be readily accessible and available to all local and state leaders, as well as the American people.

● **Direct dialogue with the American people on COVID-19 led by public health experts.** The federal government will widely distribute regular COVID updates to the general public and host regular public town halls, roundtables, and other events on COVID-19 related topics, including vaccination hesitancy. Scientists and public health and medical experts developing federal, state and local solutions will answer questions from and communicate directly with key stakeholders.

● **Build simpler, more accessible digital tools for the public.**

The federal government will improve and clarify existing COVID-19-specific websites, and will ensure that Americans can simply and easily find information relevant to them on everything from testing, vaccines, testimonials, and all available public health guidance.

Publicly share data around key response indicators. Metrics and metric-driven public health guidance will be essential to controlling the pandemic. President Biden issued Executive Order *Ensuring a Data-Driven Response to COVID-19 and Future High Consequence Public Health Threats* directing steps to enhance federal agencies' collection, production sharing, and analysis of, and collaboration with respect to, data supportive of an equitable COVID-19 response and recovery. The federal government will track a range of performance measures and targets including cases, testing, vaccinations, and hospital admissions to make real-time information readily available and inform policymakers at the federal, state, and local level. The CDC will also maintain a public dashboard tracking COVID-19 cases at the county level, so that Americans can gauge the level of transmission in their own communities to make their own informed choices.

● **Track national and state-by-state performance based on transparent, metric-driven data.** The federal government will track national and state-by-state data on a range of performance metrics including COVID-19 cases, tests, vaccinations, hospital admissions, nursing home capacity, hospital bed capacity, supply chain shortages. And the federal government will establish data systems for tracking COVID-19 outbreaks, future outbreaks across the country, and response efforts to mitigate those outbreaks. The CDC will also maintain public dashboard data at the county level on key COVID-19 related metrics. COVID-19 data with non-personally identifiable information will be open to the public and machine-readable to the maximum extent permissible to track performance, support forecasting, ensure transparency, and promote scientific research.

● **Use data to effectively communicate the state of the pandemic and drive the policy response.** Public health leaders and experts will share metrics on the state of the pandemic, drawing on existing consensus expert recommendations. These metrics and recommendations will be readily accessible for all local and state leaders, as well as the general public. The federal government will identify and communicate key metrics for understanding the pandemic and provide data that can drive response efforts and decisions; tracking a range of information including cases, testing, contact tracing, and hospitalizations to make real-time information readily usable by policymakers at different levels of government.

- **Obtain data that allows the United States to measure and evaluate the impact of response efforts in real time.** The United States will also track key metrics of success in suppressing the COVID-19 pandemic and hold regular briefings, using the best available data, to inform the American public on the current status of response efforts, evaluating pandemic response efforts using the most accurate and up-to-date data.

- **Ensure high-quality COVID-19 data is available.** Executive order *Ensuring a Data-Driven Response to COVID-19 and Future High Consequence Public Health Threats* directs steps to enhance federal agencies' ability to collect, produce, share, analyze, and collaborate in order to support COVID-19 response and recovery. The Federal Government will also work to strengthen state, local, and private sector efforts to collect COVID-19 data on a range of issues that are needed to beat the virus, including case rates, stratified by key demographics (eg race and ethnicity), cases by setting (eg LTCF, prisons and other congregate settings), hospital and ICU capacity, testing access and turn around time, effectiveness of contact tracing and quarantine efforts, and physical distancing and masking adherence..

- **Ensure state and local-level data is available to better manage the pandemic and provide support to mayors and governors deciding on COVID-19 interventions.** The federal government will support state and local governments with data personnel, technology, and other resources. This will include efforts to support transparent, interoperable data reporting from local/state and health care systems on COVID-19 and the deployment and management of data support teams to federal, state and local public health agencies that need help providing timely, reliable data to the federal government. The purpose of the coordination will be to ensure data from states and localities on common metrics are collected, aggregated, shared, analyzed, and communicated in real time to support specific public health interventions.

Engage the American people. The federal government cannot solve this crisis alone. It will take regular engagement with the public, state and local leaders, the private sector, unions, community volunteers, and health care providers to guide policy and implementation. The Administration will prioritize outreach to state and local governments, the public and private sectors, vulnerable communities, students, workers, and community leaders, using input from these stakeholders to drive the government's COVID-19 response.

- **Conduct outreach to drive the government's COVID-19 response.** The federal government will conduct outreach to the private and public sectors and communities throughout the country to begin building confidence in science and evidence-based decision-making. The goal is clear and consistent communication with the American people to address the concerns of specific communities and ensure everyone has accurate and up-to-date information.

- **Empower local community leaders to carry a science-based, public health message.** The federal government will work to identify leaders and organizations who can reach out to their communities to deliver information around vaccinations, mitigation practices, and other important public health information related to COVID-19. The Centers for Disease Control and Prevention (CDC) will provide toolkits for local leaders and state and local organizations, empowering Americans to have one-on-one conversations with friends, family members, neighbors, and members of their communities.

Lead science-first public health campaigns. The Administration will lead world-class public education campaigns — covering topics like vaccinations and vaccine hesitancy, masking, and testing — designed with diversity and inclusivity in mind, including communications in multiple languages, to maximize reach and effectiveness. The campaigns will be coordinated, across national, state, and local levels, and engage with the private and public sector. They will be anchored by science and fact-based public health guidance. The Administration will work to counter misinformation and disinformation about the safety and efficacy of the vaccine by ensuring that Americans are obtaining science-based information.

- **Encourage engagement to support the campaign.** In order to scale this public education campaign, the federal government will launch an unprecedented effort to encourage outside entities in the public and private sector to scale communication and other efforts to support vaccination and mitigation efforts. The effort will include America's leading businesses, civil rights organizations, community based organizations, foundations, health care organizations, media companies, sports leagues, tech companies, unions and COVID-19 coalitions. Organizations in every sector will be encouraged to make significant commitments toward encouraging and facilitating vaccinations and following public health guidelines.

- **Address Disinformation and Misinformation.** The federal government will develop capacity to quickly identify disinformation and misinformation and work closely with stakeholders to ensure that accurate, science-based information is available to the American people.

- **Address vaccine hesitancy especially in hard to reach communities.** The federal government's public health campaign will directly address the various reasons for COVID-19 vaccine hesitancy and combat particular types of misinformation related to vaccinations. The campaign will reach the entire U.S. population with a focus on people who may be vaccine hesitant, including rural populations and communities of color. The public health campaign will target outreach to diverse audiences and hard to reach populations.

- **Provide clear information on how people can get vaccinated.** The public health campaign will encourage vaccinations, provide factual information about vaccines, and provide clear guidance about how people can get vaccinated.

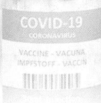

Mount a safe, effective, equitable vaccination campaign

KEY ACTIONS

— Ensure the availability of safe, effective vaccines for the American public
— Accelerate getting shots into arms and get vaccines to the communities that need them most
— Create as many venues as needed for people to be vaccinated
— Focus on hard-to-reach and high-risk populations
— Fairly compensate providers, and states and local governments for the cost of administering vaccinations.
— Drive equity throughout the vaccination campaign and broader pandemic response
— Launch a national vaccinations public education campaign
— Bolster data systems and transparency for vaccinations
— Monitor vaccine safety and efficacy
— Surge the health care workforce to support the vaccination effort

IMMEDIATE ACTIONS

The President has taken immediate action to implement goal two of the National Strategy by directing the initial actions necessary to convert vaccines into vaccinations, including improving allocation, distribution, tracking, and support to state governments.

The United States will spare no effort to ensure the public can get vaccinated quickly, effectively and equitably. To meet the aggressive vaccination target of 100 million shots by the first 100 days, the federal government will work with states and the private sector to effectively execute an aggressive vaccination strategy, focusing on the immediate actions necessary to convert vaccines into vaccinations, including improving allocation, distribution, administration, tracking, and support to State, local, Tribal and territorial governments. At the same time, the Administration will mount an unprecedented public campaign to build trust around vaccination and communicate the importance of maintaining public health measures such as masking, physical distancing, testing, and contact tracing even as people receive safe and effective vaccinations.

> " TO MEET THE AGGRESSIVE VACCINATION TARGET OF 100 MILLION SHOTS BY THE FIRST 100 DAYS, THE FEDERAL GOVERNMENT WILL WORK WITH STATES AND THE PRIVATE SECTOR TO EFFECTIVELY EXECUTE AN AGGRESSIVE VACCINATION STRATEGY, FOCUSING ON THE IMMEDIATE ACTIONS NECESSARY TO CONVERT VACCINES INTO VACCINATIONS, INCLUDING IMPROVING ALLOCATION, DISTRIBUTION, ADMINISTRATION, TRACKING, AND SUPPORT TO STATE, LOCAL, TRIBAL AND TERRITORIAL GOVERNMENTS.

This will be a whole-of-society effort that mobilizes every resource available to us — across the public and private sectors. It will take every American doing their part. And there is no one turnkey solution that works best for all. That is why this plan weaves together a strategic framework of channels designed to, together, best meet the needs of communities across the country — across ages, races, and communities large and small. And as we move forward to get vaccines in arms as quickly as possible, we will not leave anyone behind. Communities across the country are counting on it.

To mount an effective, equitable vaccination campaign, the United States will:

Ensure the availability of safe, effective vaccines for the American public. The national vaccination effort will be one of the greatest operational challenges America has ever faced. To ensure all Americans can be vaccinated quickly, the President has developed a plan for expanding vaccine manufacturing and purchasing COVID-19 vaccine doses for the U.S. population by fully leveraging contract authorities, including the Defense Production Act, deploying onsite support to monitor contract manufacturing operations, and purchasing additional FDA-authorized vaccines to deliver as quickly as possible. The effort includes prioritizing supplies that could cause bottlenecks, including glass vials, stoppers, syringes, needles, and the "fill and finish" capacity to package vaccine into vials. The plan will ensure the manufacture and purchase of sufficient supply of vaccines authorized by the FDA to vaccinate all people within the United States and Americans overseas.

- **Fill urgent gaps to spur production.** Timely vaccine production depends not only on sufficient supply of biological materials for the vaccine itself but also of appropriate equipment and materials for packaging the vaccine. Shortages of any of these materials can slow vaccine manufacturing and availability to the public. The United States will fully leverage its contracting authorities, including using the Defense Production Act, to strengthen the vaccination supply chain for raw materials and equipment and fill urgent vaccination-related supply and distribution gaps, anticipating a protracted requirement for vaccines. This will include supplies such as low-dead volume syringes with the ability to extract additional vaccine doses from vials. The Administration will also leverage all available authorities to support the expansion of lipid nanoparticle formulation capacity in order to scale mRNA vaccine production. This has implications for this pandemic as well as for the future, given the expected central role of mRNA vaccines in responding to future epidemics.

- **Deploy onsite support to monitor manufacturing operations.** Manufacturing facilities will continue to benefit from support for converting raw materials into vaccines. The federal government, through the Biomedical Advanced Research and Development Authority (BARDA), will work closely with the multitude of public and private actors involved in the end-to-end production of vaccines. The Administration will provide ongoing technical assistance and ensure that representatives are onsite at all contracted manufacturing facilities to monitor and support operations in order to support timely and effective production of vaccine supply.

- **Secure additional FDA-authorized vaccines to deliver as quickly as possible.** Especially in the early months, vaccine supply will be one of the greatest limiting factors to rapidly vaccinating the public. The United States will secure doses of FDA-authorized vaccines to deliver to the public as rapidly as possible. Timely negotiations of amendments and/or exercising supply options to existing agreements will be critical for an uninterrupted and adequate vaccine supply. The approach will center on maximizing available supply of vaccines shown to be safe and effective, while maintaining a focus on candidates that are readily manufactured, distributed and administered in support of the ultimate goal of expanding access to the entire U.S. population.

- **Continue research and development to ensure the availability of safe and effective vaccines.** The federal government will continue to support research into the use of vaccines for adolescents and children, and in the development of vaccines, formulations and delivery or administration modalities designed to minimize logistical and ancillary supply challenges. The virus will continue to evolve, with the potential for new viral strains to impact the effectiveness of existing vaccines. The United States must be able to quickly identify and understand emerging variants. To that end, the federal government, through the National Institutes of Health (NIH), the FDA, and BARDA will continue to assess the impact of emerging mutated viral strains on vaccine effectiveness, prepare to alter vaccines, if needed, and conduct vaccine research and development toward a universal or broadly acting coronavirus vaccine. The federal government will explore dose-sparing strategies that have the potential to substantially expand vaccine supply, while maintaining a commitment to abiding by FDA recommendations.

Accelerate getting shots into arms and get vaccines to the communities that need them most. To meet the aggressive vaccination target of 100 million vaccinations in the first 100 days, the United States will accelerate getting shots into arms and strengthen the distribution of vaccines to high-risk and high-need communities. In order to expand the supply available to states, the Administration will end the policy of holding back significant levels of doses, instead holding back a small reserve and monitoring supply to ensure that everyone receives the full regimen as recommended by the FDA. The Administration will also improve the allocation process by providing states and localities with clear, consistent projections to inform their planning. Critically, the United States will accelerate the pace of vaccinations by encouraging states and localities to move through the priority groups more quickly—expanding access to all individuals over the age of 65 starting in February, while staying laser-focused on ensuring that the highest-risk members of the public, including racial, ethnic and rural populations and those in congregate facilities, can access the vaccine where and when they need it. The federal government will track national and state vaccination progress, working hand-in-hand with states, immunization managers and localities to support their efforts. Through it all, the United States will work to ensure that the vaccine is distributed quickly, effectively and equitably, with a focus on high-risk groups and a commitment to provide vaccines to hard-to-reach communities.

- **Reduce federal hold back of doses to spur vaccine availability, while maintaining a commitment to the FDA-recommended two-dose schedule.** The Administration will end the policy of holding back significant levels of doses. This will accelerate the supply available now to the American public. To continue ensuring second-dose availability on the timeline recommended by the FDA, the Administration will hold back a smaller reserve, and will closely monitor development, production, and release of vaccines, and use the Defense Production Act as needed to ensure adequate supply.

- **Call on states to expand eligibility to frontline essential workers and individuals 65 years and older.** We cannot leave supply unused, or let it expire. The Administration called on states to open up eligibility beyond health care workers and long-term facilities, to include frontline essential workers like educators, first responders, grocery store employees and anyone who is 65 and older. Adults 65 and older account for 16% of the US population but 80 percent of COVID-19 deaths in the United States. As we expand eligibility to ensure that supply does not sit on shelves unused, the United States will continue to look to the CDC Advisory Committee on Immunization Practices (ACIP) framework for an equitable, effective vaccination program, and work hand-in-hand with jurisdictions to ensure that no one is left behind.

- **Strengthen the allocation process and coordinate the logistics for federal distribution of vaccine delivery.** To effectively plan and scale distribution, states and localities rely on both advanced understanding of their allocations and timely delivery of their ordered doses. Moving forward, the federal government will provide regular projections of the allocations states and localities will receive. The Administration will build on the operational plans in place to ensure the effective distribution, storage, and transit of vaccines to states, including support for maintaining or augmenting the vaccine-specific required cold chain. The Administration will also fully leverage the Defense Production Act to fill any distribution gaps, including with respect to any needed refrigeration, transportation, or storage facilities.

● **Work with vaccine manufacturers to best serve the needs of local communities.** The Administration will work with vaccine manufacturers to advance innovative approaches to vaccine packaging and shipments, such as reducing minimum shipment sizes, in order to reach rural and other underserved communities. In recognition of state and local needs, the Department of Health and Human Services (HHS) will release guidelines for redistribution within states as needed and where appropriate to ensure that jurisdictions are following all appropriate science-based guidance while providing flexibility to meet local needs where possible. HHS will also release guidance to support jurisdictions in managing waste management needs.

Create as many venues as needed for people to be vaccinated. The federal government — in partnership with state and local communities — will create as many venues for vaccination as needed in communities and settings that people trust. This includes, but is not limited to federally supported community vaccination centers, in places like stadiums and conference centers, bringing resources to state and locally operated vaccination sites in all 50 states and 14 territories, pharmacies and retail stores, federal facilities like VA hospitals, community health centers, rural health clinics, critical access hospitals, physician offices, health systems, and mobile and on-site occupational clinics.

● **Establish new, federally supported community vaccination centers across the country.** Knowing that not all states and jurisdictions may have the resources to scale vaccination at the pace this crisis demands, the National COVID-19 Response Team will utilize federal resources and emergency contracting authorities to launch new vaccination sites in support of state and local efforts to best meet local needs. The Department of Defense (DOD) will bring its logistical expertise and staff to bear, with the Federal Emergency Management Agency (FEMA) managing set-up and operations. These sites will mobilize thousands of clinical and non-clinical staff and contractors—including federal medics, Department of Agriculture (USDA) staff, Department of Veterans Affairs (VA) staff, and Public Health Service Commissioned Corps officers and DOD personnel—who will work hand-in-glove with the National Guard and state, territorial, Tribal, and local teams. These efforts will help us reach underserved communities and those that have been hit the hardest by this pandemic. By the end of February, there will be 100 federally-supported centers across the nation.

- **Bolster support for state- and local-run community vaccination clinics.** State and local public health departments will play a critical role in this vaccination effort — particularly in reaching the hardest-to-reach communities. The federal government will offer in-kind support and technical assistance for state-, local- and community-run vaccination clinics, including support for the construction and management of local sites, management of cold-chain storage and transportation, and procurement of personal protective equipment and ancillary vaccination supplies. The federal government will also provide capital assets, such as land and buildings, for state use in community vaccination efforts and assistance sourcing, procuring, stockpiling, and shipping supplies directly to sites. It will additionally provide clinical and non-clinical staff needed to support or staff community vaccination centers, including through the Army and Navy Medical Corps and work with state and local programs to support the Medical Reserve Corps. To support and advance state, local and community based efforts, HHS will release toolkits and guidance for operating and scaling different types of community vaccination centers—adaptable across various settings, from standard health clinics, to community-based sites like churches, to existing COVID-19 drive-through testing sites, to mobile clinics.

- **Leverage storefronts, including retail locations, grocers and pharmacies.** Millions of Americans turn to their local pharmacies every day for their medicines, flu shots, and much more. And nearly 90 percent of Americans live within five miles of a pharmacy, making these among the most accessible vaccination locations. The Administration will move quickly to jumpstart the effort to work directly with chain and independent pharmacies across the country to get Americans vaccinated. The program will begin within two weeks of President Biden assuming office, and expand moving forward into neighborhoods across the country so that the public can make an appointment and get their shot at their local retail and pharmacy locations.

- **Launch mobile vaccination clinics and work with rural providers.** The Administration will deploy mobile clinics to meet communities where they are, and also to offer vaccines in the most hard-to-reach communities, working with local providers, including primary care providers, to ensure that they have the resources they need to help get vaccines to the communities they serve. Through HHS agencies including the Health Resources and Services Administration (HRSA), CMS and CDC, and the Department of Veterans Affairs, the federal government will launch targeted programs to engage community health centers, rural health clinics and critical access hospitals to ensure that we can meet the needs of rural communities.

- **Launch new partnership with Federally Qualified Health Centers nationwide.** Federally Qualified Health Centers (FQHCs) serve more than 30 million patients each year—one in 11 people nationwide. Many are people of color and individuals struggling to make ends meet. Given the critical role that these providers play in their communities, the federal government, through HRSA and CDC, will launch a new program to ensure that FQHCs can directly access vaccine supply where needed. At the same time, the Administration will encourage jurisdictions to engage health centers closely in their overall jurisdictional plans. And to ensure that health centers have the resources they need to successfully launch vaccination programs, HRSA will launch a new program to provide guidance, technical assistance and other resources to prepare and engage these providers nationwide.

- **Bolster provider engagement and training.** Health care providers—including primary care doctors—will play a critical role in supporting the vaccination program nationwide. HHS, including through CDC, HRSA and CMS, will launch provider education and engagement programs to ensure that providers are able to appropriately store, handle, administer and report vaccinations so that they can best serve their patients.

- **Support state and local efforts to enlist emergency medical services and firefighters to support vaccination efforts.** Emergency medical services (EMS) personnel—first responders, emergency medical technicians, paramedics, and others—and firefighters play a critical role in their communities every day, and will be critical to supporting the vaccination effort nationwide. The federal government will support state and local government efforts to enlist EMS agencies to launch community vaccination clinics, building on their critical role and expertise in disaster relief. At the same time, the Administration will work hand-in-hand with states and localities to ensure that first responders nationwide—along with other frontline essential workers, like teachers, school staff and childcare workers, who play such a critical role in our communities every day—have access to the vaccine as quickly as possible..

- **Launch the COVID-19 Vaccinations Collaborative to support information and best practices sharing across states, localities, tribes and territories.** Vaccinating the public at the speed and scale demanded of this moment, given the requirements of the authorized vaccines, will be a first-time effort for all partners involved. Undoubtedly, given the nature of this effort, unforeseen challenges will present themselves at the state, local and provider levels. To facilitate sharing of best practices in real-time across states, localities, Tribes and territories, and to communicate clearly across all levels of government, the federal government will launch the COVID-19 Vaccinations Collaborative to provide a forum for public health leaders to directly solicit and receive feedback from peers across the nation, as well as from the federal government.

Focus on hard-to-reach and high-risk populations. As the United States accelerates the pace of vaccinations nationwide, we will remain focused on building programs to meet the needs of hard-to-reach and high-risk populations, and meeting communities where they are to make vaccinations as accessible and equitable as possible. The federal government will deploy targeted strategies to meet the needs of individuals at increased risk and others who need to take extra precautions, according to the CDC, as well as the communities hardest hit by this pandemic. Local public health will play a critical role.

- **Partner with Tribal Nations and other key entities to support an effective and equitable vaccination program.** Native Americans have been disproportionately harmed by the COVID-19 pandemic. The Biden-Harris

Administration will bolster support for Tribal Nations and Urban Indian Health Programs (UIHPs) by affirming the ability, and building the capacity, of the Indian Health Service (IHS), Tribes, Bureau of Indian Education (BIE) schools and UIHPs to provide vaccines for Native communities. The federal government will take all available steps to strengthen distribution and ordering for tribes and UIHPs. The Administration will partner with Tribal Nations to address the unique logistics and supply chain management needs in rural and remote locations and help remedy infrastructure barriers to public health in Indian country, while also supporting vaccine and public health messaging that embraces traditional practices and languages. President Biden has called on Congress to provide additional funds to the Indian Health Service to support expanded health services, address lost revenues, and support testing and vaccination efforts.

● **Launch new models to serve high-risk individuals and others who may need to take extra precautions, as identified by the CDC.** President Biden is committed to serving state and local jurisdictions in their efforts to protect those most vulnerable to the spread of COVID-19. To do so, the Administration will make models like the CDC Pharmacy Partnership for Long-Term Care Program available for other high-risk congregate settings, including homeless shelters, jails, and institutions that serve individuals with intellectual and developmental disabilities. The federal government will also work with providers to serve high-risk individuals, such as those with certain medical conditions like renal dialysis patients, including provider engagement, technical assistance and support.

● **Reach seniors in congregate settings, in the community and in their homes.** According to the CDC, older adults are at greater risk of requiring hospitalization or dying if diagnosed with COVID-19. To increase incentives to vaccinate Medicare beneficiaries, CMS will evaluate how to incorporate quality measures for COVID-19 immunizations into its value-based purchasing programs, including Medicare Advantage Star-Ratings, the physician quality payment program, and accountable care programs. Such measures would be similar to how Medicare today promotes distribution of the annual flu vaccine. CMS will also use Medicare data to identify beneficiaries at the highest-risk and work with states and localities to operationalize vaccination plans. The Administration will also build on the CDC Pharmacy Partnership for Long-Term Care (LTC) Program to ensure that long-term care residents and staff can receive vaccinations in as streamlined and effective manner as possible.

- **Distribute vaccines to facility staff and incarcerated individuals in jails, prisons and detention centers.** Incarcerated individuals and facility staff are at high risk of infection and in many cases severe illness and death due to COVID-19. These populations are disproportionately people of color. In addition to taking steps to ensure adequate mitigation measures, the federal government will move to vaccinate this population through a vaccination program run through the Bureau of Prisons and by working with states and localities to encourage the vaccination of incarcerated individuals along with facility staff as supply is available.

- **Ensure that military personnel, veterans and their families have access to vaccines.** Over 150,000 veterans under the care of Veterans Affairs (VA) have tested positive for COVID-19, with over 7,000 deaths. The VA will build on prior efforts to launch a comprehensive program to vaccinate veterans, their families and their caregivers through VA hospitals, clinics and community-based sites—ensuring that vaccination is proceeding swiftly and safely. At the same time, the Departments of State and Defense will build on their work to accelerate the pace of vaccinations for U.S. individuals overseas and military personnel, as well as locally employed staff of the U.S. Government, and their families.

- **Reach U.S. territories and freely-associated states.** An effective, equitable vaccination program will need to address the unique challenges faced by U.S. territories and freely associated states, including Puerto Rico. The federal government will expand access to cold-chain storage and strengthen the distribution and transportation process to ensure that vaccines can get to these communities effectively, equitably, and timely.

Fairly compensate providers, and states and local governments for the cost of administering vaccinations. Fairly compensating providers, and state and local governments for the costs of vaccine administration will be critical to expanding vaccination participation. President Biden will work with Congress to expand the Federal Medicaid Assistance Percentage (FMAP) to 100 percent for vaccinations of Medicaid enrollees—with the goal of alleviating state costs for administration of these vaccines and supporting states in their work to meet the needs of their communities. HHS will ask the Centers for Medicare & Medicaid Services to consider whether current payment rates for vaccine administration are appropriate or whether a higher rate may more accurately compensate providers. The federal government will fund vaccine supply and will greatly expand funding for vaccine administration by allowing state and local governments to reimburse vaccination administration expenses through the FEMA Disaster Relief Fund and by ensuring that workforce and equipment expenses for state and local-run sites are also eligible.

Drive equity throughout the vaccination campaign and broader pandemic response. The United States will drive equity in vaccinations by using demographic data to identify communities hit hardest by the virus and supporting them, ensuring no out-of-pocket costs for vaccinations, and making sure that vaccines reach those communities. Working with state, local and community-based organizations and trusted health care providers, like community health centers will be central to this effort.

- **Increase use of demographic data to identify and remedy disparities in rates of vaccination.** The United States will expand use of demographic data to identify and assist hard-hit communities — including communities of color, immigrant communities, and Indigenous and rural communities — as well as track vaccine resource distribution and evaluate vaccination campaign effectiveness.

- **Ensure no out-of-pocket costs for vaccines.** The Administration is committed to ensuring that safe, effective, cost-free vaccines are available to the entire U.S. public—regardless of their immigration status. The Secretaries of HHS, Labor, and Treasury will take action so all people in the United States — regardless of their immigration status, as well as Americans overseas — can access the vaccine free-of-charge and without cost-sharing. The Administration will ensure that providers or other entities that receive vaccine doses from the federal government may not bill patients for any expenses associated with the vaccine.

- **Address barriers to vaccination in underserved communities.** The United States will leverage federal authorities and resources to ensure distribution of the vaccine in underserved communities, including provision of convenient and accessible vaccination sites, increased clinical and community-based workforce for outreach, education and vaccination, and wrap-around supportive services. In addition, the Administration will secure commitments from the public and private sector for paid time-off, subsidized transportation costs and other incentives for those seeking to get vaccinated.

- **Encourage states to account for equity in their pandemic planning.** The federal government will request that states update their pandemic plans, as needed, to describe how they will deliver vaccines to residents at highest risk and in high-vulnerability areas using CDC's Social Vulnerability Index or another appropriate index.

Launch a national vaccinations public education campaign. The United States will build public trust through an unprecedented vaccination public health campaign at the federal, State, Tribal, territorial, local and community level. The public education campaign will support vaccination programs, address vaccine hesitancy, help simplify the vaccination process for Americans, and educate the public on effective prevention measures. The campaign will be tailored to meet the needs of diverse communities, get information to trusted, local messengers, and outline efforts to deliver a safe and effective vaccine as part of a national strategy for beating COVID-19.

- **Work with major provider associations to launch a targeted campaign to build vaccine trust.** The U.S. public trusts their health care providers to provide reliable information on the COVID-19 vaccine. The Administration will work with major provider associations— representing millions of doctors, nurses, and other health care workers nationwide—to engage providers so that they can provide detailed, accurate, and up-to-date vaccine recommendations for their patients.

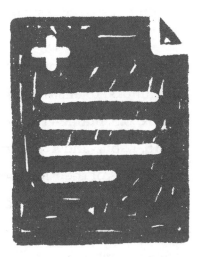

- **Build public confidence.** The Administration will highlight and build on the CDC Vaccinate with Confidence campaign to build public trust in the COVID-19 vaccines. The Administration will work with CDC and other federal partners to develop and distribute culturally-competent, multilingual public education materials. The Administration will identify campaigns aimed at delivering misinformation and disinformation to the public about the safety and efficacy of the vaccine and will work to ensure Americans are reading science-based information about the vaccine.

● **Emphasize the need to continue public health measures like masking, physical distancing, testing, tracing, and supported isolation.** Even as we ramp up vaccinations, the national public health campaign will emphasize the need to continue public health measures like masking, physical distancing, testing, tracing, and supported isolation and quarantine, in line with CDC guidance.

● **Partner with governors and State, Tribal, territorial and local health officials.** The United States will provide federal support to current state and local vaccination planning, understand and respond to the current vaccine supply gap, address and fill vaccination workforce requirements at the state and local level, and overcome challenges with vaccination prioritization, distribution, and administration planning. The President, Vice President, and the COVID-19 Response Coordinator will convene governors, mayors, Tribal and territorial leaders, public health officials, and community leaders to discuss a collaborative, unified State, local, Tribal, and territorial vaccination planning effort. The CDC will provide consistent communication and leadership with state, territorial and local health agencies to ensure that public health efforts on the ground have the resources they need.

● **Engaging with public and private sector organizations.** The Administration will ask the nation's leading businesses; civic, religious and civil rights organizations; unions; trade associations; and foundations to make unprecedented commitments to help our communities recover. These commitments will include encouraging everyone eligible to get vaccinated, and addressing barriers to vaccination like paid time off and subsidized transportation.

● **Launch a National COVID-19 Vaccination Ambassadors Program.** Recognizing the importance of trusted messengers, the Administration will launch a nationwide campaign to highlight the stories and experiences of individuals who have received the vaccine and are working in their communities to encourage others to do the same. To support this effort, and in recognition of the importance of consistent messages at the state and local levels, CDC will develop a toolkit to support communities in developing their own local ambassador programs.

- **Bring the full resources of the federal government to bear in reaching the U.S. public.** Millions of Americans depend on the U.S. Government every day—for health care, transportation, mail and other critical public services. The Administration will deploy a whole of government effort to reach the public through the federal agencies we interact with every day. For example, this includes working through the U.S. Department of Agriculture to reach food workers, WIC beneficiaries, and ranchers, the U.S. Department of Education to reach educators, college students, and school staff, the U.S. Department of Labor for the millions of essential workers nationwide. And that's only the start. From the U.S. Departments of Housing and Urban Development to the Department of Veterans Affairs to Medicare and Social Security — public services provided by the government will help carry the message about the safety and efficacy of the vaccine.

Bolster data systems and transparency for vaccinations. The operational complexity of vaccinating the public will make robust data and its use in decision-making related to vaccinations more important than ever. The federal government, with CDC, will track distribution and vaccination progress, working hand-in-hand with states and localities to support their efforts. The Administration will build on and strengthen the U.S. Government's approach to data collection related to vaccination efforts, removing impediments and developing communication and technical assistance plans for jurisdictions and providers. The Administration, through HHS and other federal partners, will rely on data to drive decision-making and the national vaccinations program.

- **Manage vaccination progress.** Data on how states are tracking against their targets and how well vaccine administration locations are reaching individuals will be critical to rapid operational enhancements. To proactively identify where states and localities may need additional support vaccinating their populations, we will track administered doses relative to allocations. Decisions on how to effectively deploy resources, and where, also rely on an understanding of what factors are driving vaccination rates. To this end the Administration will also collect information on vaccination coverage and confidence, including percentage of population vaccinated with an initial dose, percentage vaccinated with a full regimen, timeliness of regimen completion, level of vaccine confidence, and reasons for dropping out of or refusing vaccination. Finally, we will also collect information on vaccine handling, including temperature-abuse, wastage, stock-outs, and disruption in regimens due to stock-outs.

● **Strengthen data systems and provide support.** The Administration will deploy a cross-functional team of experts to partner with HHS, the CDC and other federal partners to monitor and strengthen the software systems that support our pandemic response efforts. The Administration will partner and collaborate with State, local, Tribal, territorial officials as well as providers to ensure that their experience using these systems is as effective and streamlined as possible. This will include a focus on moving to improved integrations between critical software systems and streamlining data reporting processes.

● **Ensure the security of the COVID-19 vaccination program.** The U.S. Government will counter any threat to the vaccination program. To do so, the Director of National Intelligence will lead an assessment of ongoing cyber threats and foreign interference campaigns targeting COVID-19 vaccines and related public health efforts. The U.S. Government will take steps to address cyber threats to the fight against COVID-19, including cyber attacks on COVID-19 research, vaccination efforts, the health care systems and the public health infrastructure.

Monitor vaccine safety and efficacy. The Administration will ensure that scientists are in charge of all decisions related to vaccine safety and efficacy. The FDA will also continue to honor its commitment to make relevant data on vaccine safety and efficacy publicly available and to provide opportunities for public, non-governmental expert input. Through expanded and existing systems, the CDC and FDA will ensure ongoing, real-time safety monitoring. Through it all, the Administration will communicate clearly with the American public to continue to build trust around the vaccine and its benefits for individuals, their families and communities.

Surge the health care workforce to support the vaccination effort.
A diverse, community-based health care workforce is essential to an effective vaccination program. The United States will address workforce needs by taking steps to allow qualified professionals to administer vaccines and encourage states to leverage their flexibility fully to surge their workforce, including by expanding scope of practice laws and waiving licensing requirements as appropriate.

- **Support states with federal resources.** The Administration will deploy thousands of federal staff, contractors and volunteers to support state and local vaccination efforts. This includes utilizing the U.S. Public Health Service Commissioned Corps to deliver direct clinical training and vaccination program development across the country. The effort will also use the resources of the U.S. Department of Veterans Affairs and the Department of Defense, including physicians, nurses, physician assistants, and pharmacists.

- **Fully reimburse state deployment of the National Guard.** Many states report plans to use their National Guard to support vaccine distribution efforts, including to support critical transportation and logistics functions. To further support states, the Administration will fully reimburse states for the use of their National Guard.

- **Leverage federal authorities to expand the vaccinator workforce.** The Administration will act swiftly to amend the current COVID-19 Public Readiness and Emergency Preparedness Act (PREP Act) declaration to permit certain qualified professionals (e.g. recently retired doctors and nurses) that are not licensed under state law to administer vaccines to do so in order to expand the number of qualified professionals able to administer the vaccine, with appropriate training.

- **Encourage states to surge their vaccinator workforce.** The Biden-Harris Administration will release guidance encouraging states to take all available actions to surge their workforce as appropriate, as a number of states have done. To expand medical professionals, the Administration will encourage states to consider: allowing for rapid re-licensure for health care professionals; providing temporary vaccination licenses for clinical students and foreign-educated health care professionals; and expanding scope of practice for non-physician health practitioners, including but not limited to physician assistants, pharmacists, and registered nurses.

● **Launch training, outreach and technical assistance programs.**
HHS will launch a comprehensive, agency-wide effort to provide states, localities, providers, and community-based organizations with the resources they need to mount an effective, equitable vaccination program. The program will include expert resources from CDC. As part of the effort, HRSA will launch a new training program for community health workers focused on vaccination operations and uptake to ensure that they have the resources they need to meet the needs of the communities they serve.

Mitigate spread through expanding masking, testing, treatment, data, workforce, and clear public health standards

KEY ACTIONS

— Implement masking nationwide by working with governors, mayors, and the American people
— Scale and expand testing
— Prioritize therapeutics and establish a comprehensive, integrated COVID-19 treatment discovery and development program.
— Develop actionable, evidence-based public health guidance
— Expand the U.S. public health workforce and increase clinical care capacity for COVID-19
— Improve data to guide the response to COVID-19

IMMEDIATE ACTIONS

The President has taken immediate action to implement goal three of the National Strategy by implementing masking; expanding testing; improving the public health workforce; modernizing data systems for COVID-19 and future epidemics; and providing for equitable access to treatments.

— Executive Order: Protecting the Federal Workforce and Requiring Mask-Wearing (January 20, 2021)
— Executive Order: Promoting COVID-19 Safety in Domestic and International Travel (January 21, 2021)
— Executive Order: Establishing the National Pandemic Testing Board and Ensuring a Sustainable Public Health Workforce for COVID-19 and other Biological Threats (January 21, 2021)
— Executive Order: Ensuring a Data-Driven Response to COVID-19 and Future High Consequence Public Health Threats (January, 21, 2021)
— Executive Order: Improving and Expanding Access to Care and Treatments for COVID-19 (January 21, 2021)

A comprehensive national public health effort to control the virus — even as the vaccination program ramps up — will be critical to saving lives and restoring economic activity. The federal government will partner with State, local, Tribal and territorial leaders to implement a cohesive strategy to significantly reduce the spread of COVID-19 and release clear public health guidance to the public about what to do and when, including implementing masking; expanding testing; improving the public health workforce; modernizing data systems for COVID-19 and future epidemics; and providing equitable access to treatments. The ability to quickly test, contact trace, isolate and quarantine as appropriate is a linchpin in the work to contain the virus and stop community spread. To mitigate the spread of COVID-19 through clear public health standards, the United States will:

Implement masking nationwide by working with governors, mayors, and the American people. The President has asked the American people to do what they do best: step up in a time of crisis and wear masks. He has issued Executive Order *Protecting the Federal Workforce and Requiring Mask-Wearing* which directs compliance with CDC guidance on masking and physical distancing in Federal buildings, on Federal lands, and by Federal employees and contractors. Additionally, he issued Executive Order *Promoting COVID-19 Safety in Domestic and International Travel* which directs applicable agencies to take immediate action to require mask-wearing on many airplanes, trains, and certain other forms of public transportation in the United States. He has called on governors, public health officials, mayors, business leaders, and others to implement masking, physical distancing, and other CDC public measures to control COVID-19.

- **Ask all Americans to wear masks.** President Biden has called on every American to wear a mask for 100 days when they are around people outside of their household. As of January 2021, 35 states and the District of Columbia and Puerto Rico, have mandatory masking, with remaining states never or only sometimes requiring masks. The President has called on governors and local leaders to make mask-wearing mandatory in their states and local jurisdictions and to support state mask-wearing orders where they already exist.

Statewide Mask Mandates

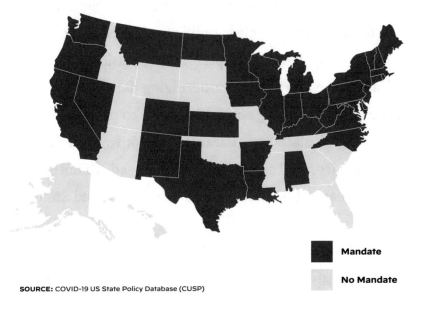

Mandate

No Mandate

SOURCE: COVID-19 US State Policy Database (CUSP)

Respondents Reporting that Community Members Wear Masks All or Most of the Time

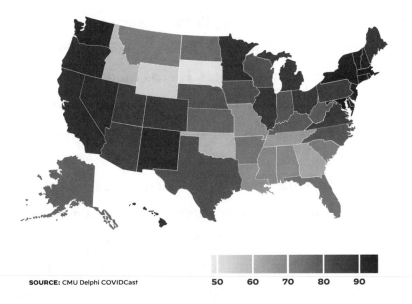

SOURCE: CMU Delphi COVIDCast

50   60   70   80   90

● **Require masking on federal property.** Executive Order *Protecting the Federal Workforce and Requiring Mask-Wearing* requires masks and specific physical distancing requirements in federal buildings, on federal lands, on military bases, and other overseas locations, consistent with CDC guidance. The Executive Order also requires ongoing guidance to ensure the safety of federal employees and directs the Centers for Disease Control and Prevention (CDC) to develop a testing plan for the federal workforce.

- **Require masking for interstate travel.** The President issued an Executive Order that directs applicable agencies to take action to require mask-wearing in airports and on certain modes of public transportation, including on many airplanes, trains, and maritime vessels, and intercity bus services.

- **Encourage adherence to masking and physical distancing.** The White House will coordinate with stakeholders and initiate an aggressive, coordinated public health campaign to encourage mask wearing, physical distancing, and following CDC guidance and other best practices. As part of the public health campaign, the federal government will step up efforts to combat misinformation and disinformation related to public health practices, including on social media platforms.

- **Promote guidance, research, and incentives for mask wearing and other public health practices.** Executive Order *Protecting the Federal Workforce and Requiring Mask-Wearing* directs agencies to identify ways to support those who implement best practices in mask wearing, physical distancing, and other CDC-recommended public health practices. The federal government will provide technical assistance and support for states who adopt model policies, and provide federal research grants to identify best practices and barriers to implementing effective masking and physical distancing policies. The CDC will also issue more detailed infection control guidance and guidance regarding mask wearing and other PPE in the workplace that is specific to different industry sectors.

- **Support businesses and others for implementing effective infection control practices.** The Small Business Administration (SBA) will provide technical support for businesses and others for implementing effective infection control practices, including administrative controls, engineering controls, and PPE. The SBA will also work to develop incentives to encourage small businesses to adopt adequate infection control practices including effective and enforced mask wearing policies and other social distancing policies.

● **Provide resources to schools that sign up for appropriate mask wearing, physical distancing and testing policies.** The federal government will support and provide resources to schools that sign up for appropriate mask wearing, physical distancing, and testing policies.

Scale and expand testing. To control the COVID-19 pandemic and safely reopen schools and businesses, America must have wide-spread testing. A national testing strategy is a cornerstone to reducing the spread of COVID-19 and controlling outbreaks, and clear Federal guidance and a unified national approach to implementation are essential. Executive Order *Protecting the Federal Workforce and Requiring Mask-Wearing* establishes the COVID-19 Pandemic Testing Board to oversee implementation of a clear, unified approach to testing. The United States will expand the rapid testing supply and double test supplies and increase testing capacity. The United States will also increase onshore test manufacturing, enhance laboratory capacity to conduct testing over the short- and long-term, stand up a CDC Testing Support Team, support COVID-19 screening for schools and other priority populations, work to ensure that tests are widely available, clarify health insurers' obligation to cover testing, and ensure that testing is free of charge for those who lack health insurance.

Testing Trends

April 2020 - January 2021

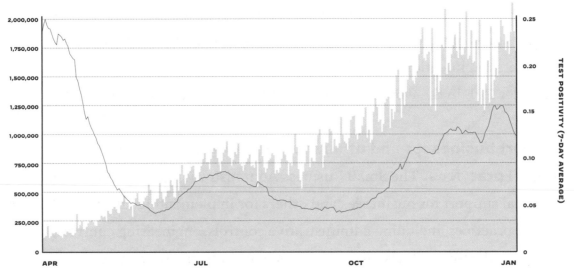

Source: COVID Tracking Project

● **Stand up the COVID-19 Pandemic Testing Board.** The COVID-19 Pandemic Testing Board–a federal interagency group chaired by the COVID-19

Response Testing Coordinator–will coordinate and oversee a clear, unified, and equitable approach to testing to be implemented across government and in partnership with states and localities and working with the private sector..

- **Surge the manufacture and production of tests.** The federal government will work to expand the production of tests and make a commitment toward a 5 year investment in the onshore manufacturing of test kits and related supplies for COVID-19 and emerging biological threats. The availability and allocation of tests, as well as test processing capacity, has been a clear barrier to containing COVID-19.

- **Expand laboratory capacity and surveillance for hotspots and variants.** The federal government seeks to invest in laboratory capacity, including long-term regional testing capacity to improve testing timelines.

- **Increasing surveillance for variants and emerging threats.** The Administration will also expand surveillance and genomic sequencing to monitor for COVID-19 hotspots, variants of concern and emerging infectious disease threats.

- **Fill testing supply shortfalls.** The federal government will exercise legal authorities, including the Defense Production Act, to expand capacity in manufacturing of tests and the supplies related to testing. The United States will also maximize production of different types of testing and create incentives for the private sector to develop, innovate, and expand testing capabilities.

- **Strengthen testing supply chain by promoting predictable and robust federal purchasing of testing supplies.** The federal government will seek to expand existing contracts, fund advance purchase agreements, and set targets for testing supply and use in settings such as schools, long-term care facilities and underserved areas. Supply constraints have been a barrier to the adoption of more wide-scale testing, particularly screening testing of individuals without known exposure. More predictable and robust federal purchasing of testing supplies will help to advance the pipeline.

- **Effectively distribute tests and expand access to testing.** The federal government will support school screening testing programs to help schools that can reopen do so. The Administration will also stand up a dedicated CDC

Testing Support Team, fund rapid test acquisition and distribution for priority populations, and work to spur development and manufacturing of at-home tests.

- **Maximize accessibility through free testing.** President Biden issued Executive Order *Establishing the National Pandemic Testing Board and Ensuring a Sustainable Public Health Workforce for COVID-19 and Other Biological Threats* directing agencies to facilitate testing free of charge for those who lack health insurance and to clarify insurers' obligation to cover testing.

- **Provide testing protocols, adequate funding and technical assistance.** The federal government will provide testing protocols to inform the use of testing in congregate settings, schools, and other critical areas and among asymptomatic individuals. Further, technical assistance would support more widespread adoption of testing to improve timely diagnosis and public confidence in the safety of settings like schools.

- **Conduct research and promote innovation in testing, including at-home tests and instant tests, to scale up America's testing capacity.** The United States will promote research and innovation in testing, including to help maximize laboratory capacity and reduce time and costs associated with COVID-19 testing. The federal government will also promote research and implementation regarding the use of surveillance testing to identify areas at high-risk for disease transmission and to inform more targeted use of existing diagnostic tools.

Prioritize therapeutics and establish a comprehensive, integrated COVID-19 treatment discovery and development program. Effective treatments for COVID-19 are critical to saving lives. The federal government will establish a comprehensive, integrated, and coordinated preclinical drug discovery and development program, with diverse clinical trials, to allow therapeutics to be evaluated and developed rapidly in response to COVID-19 and other pandemic threats. This includes promoting the immediate and rapid development of therapeutics that respond to COVID-19 by developing new antivirals directed against the coronavirus family, accelerating research and support for clinical trials for therapeutics in response to COVID-19 with a focus on those that can be readily scaled and administered, and developing broad-spectrum antivirals to prevent future viral pandemics. President Biden issued Executive Order *Improving and Expanding Access to Care and Treatment* *for COVID-19* which also outlines steps to bolster clinical care capacity, provide assistance to long-term care facilities and intermediate care facilities for people with disabilities, increase health care workforce capacity, expand access to programs designed to meet long-term health needs of patients recovering from COVID-19, and support access to safe and effective COVID-19 therapies and for those without coverage.

- **Promote immediate and rapid development of therapeutics that respond to COVID-19.** The United States will immediately accelerate research and support for clinical trials for therapeutics in response to COVID-19 with a focus on those that can be readily scaled and administered. To do so, the federal government will establish a comprehensive, integrated, and coordinated preclinical drug discovery and development program, with diverse clinical trials, to facilitate the rapid evaluation and development of therapeutics in response to COVID-19 and other future pandemic threats. As part of this program, the federal government will stand up a program to develop antivirals directed against the coronavirus family. By identifying targets (such as proteases and polymerases) that are common to all members of this virus family—which includes SARS, MERS, and SARS-CoV-2—broad-spectrum drug therapies can be developed and tested under a more expedited time frame.

- **Develop basic preclinical tools required to develop new antivirals directed against the coronavirus family.** To establish the COVID-19 therapeutics program, the federal government will facilitate and support: assay (drug testing system) development for each target; high throughput screening of currently approved drugs and collections of novel chemical starting points for each anti-infectious drug target; lead identification through medicinal chemistry to refine the molecules and improve their chances of success; in vitro and in vivo testing; pharmacokinetics and toxicology testing; chemistry, manufacturing, and controls; as well as all the regulatory work required to generate an Investigational New Drug application to the FDA, and completion of early phase clinical trials.

- **Develop broad-spectrum antivirals and prioritize other viral classes that present emerging threats to prevent future viral pandemics.** The federal government will promote the ongoing discovery and development of antivirals with broad-spectrum activity against coronaviruses, which would potentially enable rapid preclinical testing and clinical trials if and when a new zoonotic coronavirus appears. As the program unfolds, other viral classes that represent emerging pandemic threats will also be prioritized to generate new therapeutics.

● **Promote effective therapeutics that respond to COVID-19 and future pandemics by supporting and strengthening each phase of development.** The federal government will expedite and promote the development of effective therapeutics by supporting and strengthening each phase of therapeutic development. This will involve establishing and coordinating a partnership of scientists from multiple government agencies, academic institutions, industry, and professional organizations that will:

> ➋ Identify and prioritize the best therapeutic targets for inhibiting potential future viral threats
>
> ➋ Design high-throughput screening assays
>
> ➋ Facilitate the systematic testing of all antivirals in combination
>
> ➋ Complete investigational new drugIND enabling studies of potential therapeutic agents
>
> ➋ Proceed through animal model supply and testing, preclinical therapy development, early clinical therapy development
>
> ➋ Make data available as soon as possible

● **Accelerate research and development in COVID-19 treatments that addresses populations at increased risk of serious complications as a result of COVID-19.** The federal government will ensure that therapeutics development work also will include supporting emerging therapeutics research that addresses the needs of communities of color, children, pregnant women, and populations at increased risk of serious complications as a result of COVID-19, as well as directing the development of an evidence base around the long-term health impacts of COVID-19.

● **Improve access to high-quality treatments and strengthen health care services, while addressing affordability.** The United States will improve the availability of treatments and reduce the potential for therapeutics supply shortages by investing in expanded capacity through advanced manufacturing, making advanced purchases of promising therapeutics and other treatments, and strengthening data infrastructure and surveillance systems to prevent and address shortages.

Develop actionable, evidence-based public health guidance. The Centers for Disease Control and Prevention (CDC) will develop and update public health guidance on containment and mitigation that provides metrics for measuring and monitoring the incidence and prevalence of COVID-19 in health care facilities, schools, workplaces, and the general public, including metric-driven reopening guidance that the federal government communicates widely. Informed by up-to-date national and state data, the CDC will provide and update guidance on key issues such as physical distancing protocols, testing, contact tracing, reopening schools and businesses, and masking. The CDC also will provide focused guidance for older Americans and others at higher risk, including people with disabilities.

- **Develop a broad range of guidance and strategies to promote the adoption of the guidance.** CDC will issue more detailed guidance addressed to the specific needs and concerns of vulnerable populations, including older Americans and others at high-risk.

- **Elevate state model policies.** The White House, together with relevant Departments and Agencies, will convene State, local, Tribal, and territorial health leaders to develop plans and share best practices for masking, physical distancing, testing, vaccinations, and distributing PPE and other supplies. The Administration will highlight model policies for states, and provide technical support to help states with implementation of identified best practices.

- **Continue aggressive research to identify best practices for, and barriers to, implementing CDC public health guidance.** The federal government will continue to aggressively promote scientific research to identify best practices for implementing public health guidance, as well as recommendations to overcome barriers to implementation.

Expand the U.S. public health workforce and increase clinical care capacity for COVID-19. The United States must build and support an effective public health workforce to fight COVID-19 and the next public health threat. As part of the President's commitment to provide 100,000 COVID-19 contact tracers, community health workers, and public health nurses, the United States will establish a U.S. Public Health Jobs Corps, provide support for community health workers, and mobilize Americans to support communities most at-risk. The United States will also provide technical support for testing, contact tracing, vaccinations and other urgent public health workforce needs to better prepare for public health crises.

- ● **Increase clinical care capacity.** Through Executive Order *Improving and Expanding Access to Care and Treatment for COVID-19* the President has outlined immediate steps for targeted deployment of federal assets, workforce, and facilities to states to bolster critical care capacity in hotspots. The Executive Order encourages states and providers to take all available actions to support and expand the health care workforce to address staff shortages, and increases access to programs that meet the long-term health needs of patients recovering from COVID-19 through technical assistance and support to community health centers. The federal government will also take steps to bolster doctors, nurses, and other health care workers through the rapid deployment of licensed medical reservists, including active duty military and National Guard, retired providers, as well as current federal clinical workforce, including the U.S. Public Health Service Commissioned Corps.

State Representative Estimate for % of Inpatient Beds Occupied by COVID-19 Patients

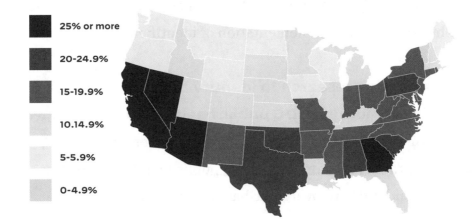

25% or more
20-24.9%
15-19.9%
10.14.9%
5-5.9%
0-4.9%

- ● **Surge 100,000 COVID-19 contact tracers, community health workers, and public health nurses.** The United States has committed to working with governors, mayors, Tribal leaders, public health officials, unions, and community organizations, to provide 100,000 COVID-19 contact tracers, community health workers, and public health nurses, taking into account the need to hire a workforce that reflects the communities where people will work. The Administration will review state contact tracing efforts, including states leading on contact tracing technologies, to scale successful programs nationally.

- ● **Leverage existing public health and training programs.** The United States will draw on existing federal programs to stand up a national contact tracing and COVID-19 public health workforce training program to hire and train public health workers for contact tracing and mass vaccination. The Biden-Harris Administration will leverage workers at the Department of Health and Human Services (HHS), CDC, FEMA, and the Department of Defense (DOD) that could assist or train state and local contact tracers, case managers, and/or vaccinators—including experienced, existing federal personnel.

Improve data to guide the response to COVID-19. Federal agencies will make increased use of data to guide the public health response against COVID-19. To that end, Agencies will collect, aggregate, share, and analyze non-personally identifiable data, and take steps to make it publicly available and in a machine-readable form to enhance COVID-19 response efforts. And the United States will support evidence-based decision-making through focused data-based projects. These efforts will require collaboration with State, local, Tribal and territorial governments to aggregate and analyze data for critical decisions to track access to vaccines and testing, reopen schools and businesses, address disparities in COVID-19 infections and health outcomes, and enhance critical monitoring capacity where needed. In addition, critical response activities such as workforce mobilization and vaccination appointment scheduling may require new technology solutions. The United States will provide technical support to ensure that these systems meet mission critical requirements to support a robust response.

- ● **Strengthen essential data systems.** The scale of the COVID-19 pandemic in the United States requires improved data systems that can manage large volumes of data, and connect with legacy and new data systems created in response to the current crisis. Critical response activities such as workforce mobilization and vaccination appointment scheduling may require new technology solutions. The United States will provide technical support to ensure that these systems meet mission critical requirements to support a robust response.

- **Directs relevant federal agencies to collect, produce, share, analyze, and collaborate with respect to data supportive of COVID-19 response and recovery efforts.** Executive Order *Ensuring a Data-Driven Response to COVID-19 and Future High Consequence Public Health Threats* directs federal agencies across government to collect, produce, share and analyze data and collaborate with respect to COVID-19 response and recovery efforts. Making appropriate protections for privacy, the COVID-19 Response Team will work to ensure that data with non-personally identifiable information is open to the public and machine-readable to the maximum extent permissible to support performance tracking and forecasting, ensure transparency, and promote scientific research.

- **Identify common federal metrics for tracking COVID-19 incidence, testing, contact tracing, hospital capacity and preparedness and treatment.** Currently, states and cities across the United States are using and reporting on different metrics. The federal government will call on states to report on a key set of common metrics, in order to determine when progress is being made and where additional resources and federal attention should be directed.

- **Assist localities that struggle with public health infrastructure challenges that limit effective reporting or managing of COVID-19 data.** The federal government will focus on states and localities that continue to struggle with antiquated data systems, especially jurisdictions that have trouble connecting testing laboratories and public health agencies to support case investigation, contact tracing, and support services for isolation of potentially exposed individuals. The federal government will work to surge personnel to assist with manual processes in the near-term and develop data technologies to automate in the long-term.

Immediately expand emergency relief and exercise the Defense Production Act

KEY ACTIONS

- Increase emergency funding to states and bolster the FEMA response
- Fill supply shortfalls by invoking the Defense Production Act
- Identify and solve urgent COVID-19 related supply gaps and strengthen the supply chain.
- Secure the pandemic supply chain and create a manufacturing base in the United States
- Improve distribution and expand availability of critical materials.

IMMEDIATE ACTIONS

The President has taken immediate action to implement goal four of the National Strategy by: strengthening the pandemic supply chain; directing immediate action to use all available legal authorities, including the Defense Production Act for PPE, testing supplies, and supplies for vaccination, and increasing federal reimbursement for states to 100% for National Guard personnel and emergency supplies, including for schools.

- Presidential Memorandum: Extend Federal Support to Governors' Use of National Guard to Respond to COVID-19 and to Increase Reimbursement and other Assistance Provided to States (January 21, 2021)
- Executive Order: A Sustainable Public Health Supply Chain (January 21, 2021)

Ensuring the availability of COVID-19-related supplies is a critical component of the government's COVID response and pandemic preparedness strategy. To date, the United States has experienced a number of supply shortages in pandemic response resources, from personal protective equipment (PPE) (e.g., masks, gloves, gowns, etc.), testing equipment and supplies (e.g., tests, reagents, nasal swabs, etc.), and medical equipment (e.g., ventilators). States have entered into regional compacts to address supply shortages and have been forced to compete with one another and the federal government to secure supplies.

This map displays a breakdown by state showing where the 19,700+ PPE requests have come from since March 2020. Get US PPE has recieved requests for PPE from all 50 states and some US territories

The map displays a breakdown by state showing where the 19,700+ PPE requests have come from since March 2020. Get Us PPE has received requests for PPE from all 50 states and some US territories.

While in some places shortages are not as acute as they were in the spring 2020, there are still hospital workers, doctors' offices, and first responders, especially in disadvantaged and Tribal communities, that cannot get regular access to the equipment they need to protect themselves while they are helping others. And even more so, critical workers such as educators and many in the food services and critical manufacturing sectors are also unable to access adequate protective equipment. Many critical workers continue to work under emergency PPE conservation rules, reusing equipment much more than is safe, and in some cases, using equipment manufactured to foreign standards that are much lower than standards in the United States.

The development of new test protocols, vaccines, and treatments will only intensify the needs for supplies. If the federal government does not act, shortages are expected to continue, especially in light of the lean nature of supply chains and the intense global competition for the same supplies.

It's time to fix America's supply shortage problems for good. To respond to this unprecedented operational challenge, the President is immediately expanding emergency relief by giving state and local governments the support they need. To ensure the availability of vaccines, tests, PPE, and other critical supplies for the duration of the pandemic, the President has directed the use of the Defense Production Act, instructing departments and agencies to fill supply shortfalls immediately for tests, personal protective equipment, therapeutics, and vaccines. The federal government will also address urgent supply gaps by coordinating, monitoring and strengthening supply chains; prioritizing essential equipment, medications, and protective gear; while also steering the distribution of supplies to areas with the greatest need.

To expand emergency relief and strengthen the supply chain, the federal government will:

Increase emergency funding to states and bolster the Federal Emergency Management Agency (FEMA) response. The President has issued a Presidential Memorandum, *Extend Federal Support to Governors' Use of National Guard to Respond to COVID-19 and to Increase Reimbursement and other Assistance Provided to States*, directing FEMA to fully reimburse states for the cost of National Guard personnel and emergency supplies, including emergency supplies like PPE for schools and child care providers.

- **Increase assistance to State, Local, and Tribal Governments for Emergency Supplies.** The President has directed FEMA to increase assistance to State, Tribal and local governments by reimbursing 100 percent of the cost of emergency supplies, which includes PPE and cleaning supplies for schools.

- **Provide 100% cost reimbursement for use of National Guard.** The President has directed FEMA to provide 100% cost reimbursement for governors' use of National Guard personnel to assist with the COVID-19 pandemic response and has also directed FEMA to consider methods for expediting payments.

● **Establish clear federal leadership.** Clear federal leadership will be essential to working with departments and agencies to ensure that there is sufficient PPE, tests, vaccines, and related supplies and equipment. The COVID-19 Response Supply Coordinator will coordinate the federal effort focused on securing, strengthening, and ensuring a sustainable pandemic supply chain.

● **Coordinate federal agencies under a unified, national Pandemic supply process.** The Supply Coordinator will coordinate the wide range of Federal agencies involved in acquisition, supply, industrial base expansion activity, and Defense Production Act activities under a single national Pandemic Supply process, ensuring synchronised efforts and demonstrating the administration's intent to use all available authorities, including contracts, purchase commitments, and investments to strengthen supply chains.

● **Engage state leaders and manufacturers and communicate the federal government's approach to supplies.** The federal government and the Supply Coordinator will prioritize the engagement of state leaders and manufacturers to communicate the federal approach to supplies, as transparency and a shared understanding of the status of existing supply efforts will be critical. And the COVID-19 Response Supply Coordinator will reduce opacity of the market for critical supplies and supply chains by clearly and rapidly communicating with states, health care providers, and manufacturers about federal interventions.

Fill supply shortfalls by invoking the Defense Production Act (DPA).
The United States is taking immediate action to fill supply shortfalls for vaccination supplies, testing supplies, and PPE. The President issued Executive Order *A Sustainable Public Health Supply Chain* which directs agencies to fill supply shortfalls using all available legal authorities, including the Defense Production Act, and the United States has identified twelve immediate supply shortfalls that will be critical to the pandemic response. The President has directed relevant agencies to exercise all appropriate authorities, including the DPA, to accelerate manufacturing, delivery, and administration to meet shortfalls in these twelve categories of critical supplies, including taking action to increase the availability of supplies like N95 masks,

isolation gowns, nitrile gloves, polymerase chain reaction (PCR) sample collection swabs, test reagents, pipette tips, laboratory analysis machines for PCR tests, high-absorbency foam swabs, nitrocellulose material for rapid antigen tests, rapid test kits, low dead-space needles and syringes, and all the necessary equipment and material to accelerate the manufacture, delivery, and administration of COVID-19 vaccine.

Scientists, researchers, and clinical trial participants have done incredible work developing multiple successful vaccines in record time. But every day longer it takes to get the population inoculated means more Americans lost. The federal government will use all authorities at its disposal to make as much vaccine as possible as quickly as possible. It is a complex process, with custom, one-of-a kind equipment to make lipid nanoparticles and handle complex chemical reactions, and all of the critical materials needed to make hundreds of millions of doses. The federal government will help make those more of these machines where possible, as well as more of the filters and vessel liners and tubing needed to speed production.

- **Use the full power of the Defense Production Act to accelerate the manufacture, delivery and administration of the COVID-19 vaccine.** On January 21, the President announced that the Administration will use the full power of the Defense Production Act and all other available legal authorities to respond to shortfalls of all necessary equipment and material to accelerate the manufacture, delivery and administration of the COVID-19 vaccine. This includes shortages in the dead-space needle syringes available to administer the Pfizer vaccine. Additional actions to utilize the Defense Production Act and other efforts to support the manufacture, delivery and administration of vaccines are detailed in National Strategy for the COVID-19 Response Goal Two: Mount a safe, effective, equitable vaccination campaign.

- **Use the full power of the Defense Production Act to respond to shortfalls in PPE.** The President directed the Administration to begin to exercise the Defense Production Act authority as needed to respond to PPE shortfalls, including U.S. made N95 Respirator and surgical masks.

- **Use the full power of the Defense Production Act to respond to shortfalls in testing.** On January 21, the President announced that the Administration will begin to exercise the Defense Production Act and all other available legal authorities to respond to testing shortfalls, including the foam swabs needed for COVID-19 rapid, point-of-care antigen tests, where results can be read within 15 minutes.

● **Use the full power of the Defense Production Act to significantly increase testing availability and decrease state-to-state competition for supplies through loans to manufacturers.** The Administration will begin to exercise Defense Production Act authority to offer attractive loans to manufacturers to dramatically increase capacity in the production of COVID-19 tests, expand testing availability, and decrease state-to-state competition for scarce supplies.

● **Continue to exercise the Defense Production Act where needed to alleviate shortfalls in vaccinations, testing, PPE, and other critical supplies.** The federal government is committed to continuing to use the DPA where needed to fill urgent vaccination-related supplies, testing, and PPE shortfalls.

Identify and solve urgent COVID-19 related supply gaps and strengthen the supply chain. Executive Order *A Sustainable Public Health Supply Chain* also directs federal agencies to fill supply shortfalls using all available legal authorities.The federal government will focus on the near-term goal of building a stable, secure, and resilient supply chain with increased domestic manufacturing in four key critical sectors:

  ➋ Antigen and molecular-based testing;
  ➋ Personal protective equipment and durable medical equipment;
  ➋ Vaccine development and manufacturing; and
  ➋ Therapeutics and key drugs.

The federal government will immediately focus on procuring supplies that will be critical to control the spread of COVID-19 by initiating contracts, entering into purchase commitments, making investments to produce supplies and expanding manufacturing capacity.

● **Conduct an immediate end-to-end inventory of vaccination supplies, testing supplies, and PPE to respond to identified shortfalls.**The federal government will identify, inventory, and monitor the need, availability, and manufacturing capacity of critical supplies. Executive Order *A Sustainable Public*

Health Supply Chain directs the federal government to conduct an immediate end-to-end inventory of major COVID-19 response supplies. This is a crucial first step to addressing U.S. pandemic and medical supply chain issues. This inventory will drive decisions about the scope, contracting, and replenishing of the Strategic National Stockpile (SNS), use of the Defense Production Act, budget requests, investments in manufacturing, decisions about prioritizing supply distribution, and commitments to the global COVID-19 response.

- **Initiate contracts, enter into purchase commitments, and make investments necessary to close critical supply gaps and meet urgent supply needs.** Where shortfalls in inventory and capacity are identified, the President has directed federal action using all available means, including the Defense Production Act authority, to initiate contracts, enter into purchase commitments, and make investments necessary to close critical supply gaps and meet urgent supply needs.

Secure the pandemic supply chain and create a manufacturing base in the United States. To respond more effectively to this crisis, and ensure that the United States is able to respond more quickly and efficiently to the next pandemic, we need a resilient, domestic public health industrial base. The U.S. Government will not only secure supplies for fighting the COVID-19 pandemic, but also build toward a future, flexible supply chain and expand an American manufacturing capability where the United States is not dependent on other countries in a crisis.

- **Develop a Pandemic Supply Chain Resilience Strategy.** The President issued Executive Order *A Sustainable Public Health Supply Chain* that directs the development of a Pandemic Supply Chain Resiliency Strategy to design, build, and sustain both a short-term and long-term capability in the United States to manufacture pandemic supplies for COVID-19 as well as the manufacture of supplies for future pandemic and biological threats. The Pandemic Supply Chain Resiliency Strategy will address onshoring production of COVID-19 and related pandemic and medical supplies, creating a manufacturing base in the United States that can fill the Strategic National Stockpile, avoiding reliance on other countries for lifesaving medicines and supplies, and allowing the speed and flexibility required to produce needed supplies and medicines for ongoing COVID-19 outbreaks and future biological crises.

- **Use the Defense Production Act to develop domestic manufactucturing of critical pandemic supplies.** Through the use of purchase agreements, loans, and other mechanisms the federal government will build additional domestic manufacturing capacity for both equipment like PPE and testing as well as reserve vaccine production lines to ensure availability of supply when we need it.

- **Enhance the nation's ability to develop, manufacture, and authorize successful vaccines built on 21st-century technologies.** The federal government will invest in state-of-the-art vaccine manufacturing facilities, accelerate clinical vaccine candidate development for priority viral pathogens, and build a stockpile of essential raw materials and ancillary supplies for vaccines.

- **Identify opportunities to invest in communities suffering from the economic impact of the pandemic.** The federal government will also work with state and local leaders to identify opportunities to invest in domestic manufacturing in communities that bear the brunt of the economic impact of COVID-19.

- **Assess plans to refill the Strategic National Stockpile to ensure preparedness for continued COVID-19 outbreaks.** The federal government will reexamine the strategic objectives and core concept of operations of the Strategic National Stockpile, as well as the resulting size and content of the reserves that will be required moving forward.

Improve distribution and expand availability of critical materials. After conducting a review of existing COVID-19 and related pandemic supply chain distribution plans and working in consultation with state and regional compacts, the United States will coordinate distribution plans, prioritizing areas of highest-risk and highest need, and set up a structure to improve the distribution of critical materials. To work toward expanding the affordability and accessibility of supplies, Executive Order *A Sustainable Public Health Supply Chain* directs DOD, HHS and DHS to develop recommendations to address the pricing of COVID-19 supplies. The federal government will also reduce the opacity of the market for critical supplies and supply chains by clearly and rapidly communicating with states, health care providers, and manufacturers about federal interventions.

- **Improve supply chain surveillance and data systems and develop tools to better assess inventory and supply needs.** The federal government will improve the resilience of pandemic-related supply chains by establishing better supply chain surveillance and data systems and improving channels of communications to assess inventory and supply needs. Additionally, the federal government will also establish and maintain mechanisms to share information to link supply deficits to rapid action procurement, manufacturing, and distribution. Resolving urgent gaps in supply will require close monitoring of supply chains for products like swabs, reagents, glass vials, and refrigeration equipment for vaccine storage and transport, while also steering distribution of supplies to areas with the greatest need.

- **Coordinate distribution to areas of need.** The federal government will work with Governors to determine their needs, coordinate production and delivery of supply to meet those needs in a timely and efficient manner; and direct the distribution of critical equipment as COVID-19 cases peak at different times in states or territories. The federal government will establish clear channels for distribution of supplies to stakeholders, using existing national, state and local infrastructure, and ensuring the equitable distribution of supplies to vulnerable populations, with a focus on communities and populations disproportionately affected by COVID-19.

- **Provide adequate testing and PPE for all medical personnel, first responders, and essential government and private-sector service providers.** The federal government will work to replenish depleted supplies in hard-hit, high-risk, and high-need areas and populations, ensuring the affordability and the availability of supplies to key groups including states, schools, workers, health care providers and facilities, and work toward bolstering availability so that users can return to the National Institute for Occupational Safety and Health single-use guidelines; while keeping the dramatic price inflation of critical items under control.

- **Identify and take steps to limit price gouging and promote reasonable pricing.** Where possible, federal commitments to contract for or invest in the manufacture of pandemic-related supplies should include measures to ensure that supplies are available at a reasonable price. The federal government will take a strong stance against price gouging and fraud. The President issued an Executive Order that directs agencies to develop recommendations for furthering the goal of reasonable pricing for COVID-19 supplies.

Safely Reopen Schools, Businesses, And Travel While Protecting Workers

KEY ACTIONS

— Implement a national strategy to support safely reopening schools
— Support safe operations at child care centers and at-home providers
— Support equitable reopening in higher education
— Protect workers and issue stronger worker safety guidance
— Provide guidance and support to safely open businesses
— Promote safe travel

IMMEDIATE ACTIONS

The President has taken immediate action to implement goal five of the National Strategy by directing immediate steps to support the safe operation of schools, businesses, and travel by giving schools the tools and resources to reopen, supporting childcare, supporting businesses to stay open safely, and reopening travel.

— Executive Order: Supporting the Reopening and Continuing Operation of Schools and Early Childhood Education Providers (January 21, 2021)
— Executive Order: Protecting Worker Health and Safety (January 21, 2021)
— Executive Order: Promoting COVID-19 Safety in Domestic and International Travel (January 21, 2021)

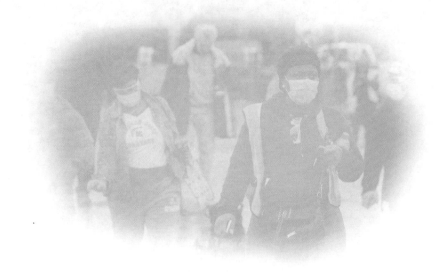

For nearly a year, communities have been hobbled by the closure of key pieces of their economic and social infrastructure. The majority of schools have been shuttered, and others have closed and opened sporadically with changes in concerns about COVID-19's spread and a lack of clear, consistent, data-driven guidance and best practices for safely keeping schools open. Schools have also suffered from a lack of available testing and other resources to operate safely. Many businesses that have complied with public health orders have suffered crippling losses of income, while others have put their employees at risk by remaining open without proper safety precautions. Some businesses, like childcare providers, have struggled to remain open safely throughout the pandemic, risking themselves in order to support the broader pandemic response, including caring for the children of first responders.

> **MANY BUSINESSES THAT HAVE COMPLIED WITH PUBLIC HEALTH ORDERS HAVE SUFFERED CRIPPLING LOSSES OF INCOME, WHILE OTHERS HAVE PUT THEIR EMPLOYEES AT RISK BY REMAINING OPEN WITHOUT PROPER SAFETY PRECAUTIONS.**

It doesn't have to be this way. The Biden-Harris Administration will direct a whole-of-government effort to ensure that schools and businesses that can open safely have the resources to do so - and that those that must remain closed have the support to do that too. It will implement safety standards for transportation and promote safe international travel. Safely reopening schools, businesses, travel, and our economy starts with doing the things we know will work to drive down COVID-19 rates and keep people safe, including masking, regular testing, and vaccination. At the same time that the United States takes these steps to decrease COVID-19 spread, it will also support safe operation of schools, businesses, and travel through major, unified federal actions to expand rapid testing, ensure a strong supply of protective gear, build a rapid response public health workforce, offer clear guidance and protections, and provide support for people to stay home when they need to.

To protect workers, safely reopen schools and businesses, and promote safe travel, the United States will:

Implement a national strategy for safely reopening schools. The United States is committed to ensuring that children and students are able to resume safe, in-person learning and care as quickly as possible. COVID-19 has been devastating for students and their families. Students have lost months of learning as a result of school closures, and losses are particularly acute for lower-income students and students of color.

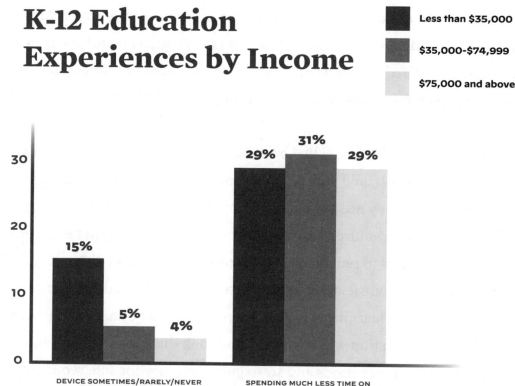

K-12 Education Experiences by Income

- Less than $35,000
- $35,000-$74,999
- $75,000 and above

DEVICE SOMETIMES/RARELY/NEVER AVAILABLE FOR EDUCATION: 15%, 5%, 4%

SPENDING MUCH LESS TIME ON LEARNING ACTIVITIES VS. PRIOR YEAR: 29%, 31%, 29%

EXECUTIVE ORDER ISSUED

The President issued Executive Order *Supporting the Reopening and Continuing Operation of Schools and Early Childhood Education Providers* which lays out a national strategy for safely reopening schools, postsecondary institutions, and early childhood education providers.

Given the disastrous impact of school closures on families, the economy and our society, it is a national priority to reopen our schools and keep them open. The Administration has set the goal of safely reopening a majority of K-8 schools in 100 days. Meeting that goal will require a comprehensive national effort to provide necessary funding, to put in place strong public health measures that we all follow, and to support school districts to adopt measures that keep students and staff safe.

The President issued Executive Order *Supporting the Reopening and Continuing Operation of Schools and Early Childhood Education Providers* which lays out a national strategy for safely reopening schools, postsecondary institutions, and early childhood education providers. The order requires the Departments of Education (ED) and Health and Human Services (HHS) to provide guidance and resources to support schools, colleges, and child care providers in safely reopening and operating. The President also issued a Presidential Memorandum *Extend Federal Support to Governors' Use of National Guard to Respond to COVID-19 and to Increase Reimbursement and other Assistance Provided to States* restoring full reimbursement for eligible costs necessary to support safe school reopening through the FEMA Disaster Relief Fund.

In addition, President Biden has called on Congress to provide $130 billion in dedicated funding to support schools, and additional resources for COVID-19 testing, so that schools have the funds they need to support reopening. This includes implementing regular COVID-19 testing, addressing transportation and ventilation needs, providing PPE hiring more teachers to reduce class sizes to allow for social distancing, hiring nurses, providing more counselors to address students' social and emotional needs, and providing additional learning supports for students (like summer school or tutoring). The Administration will release a handbook that helps schools and local leaders implement the precautions and strategies necessary for safe reopening. It will also work with states and local school districts to support screening testing in schools, including working to ensure an adequate supply of test kits and providing

> **"IN THE COMING WEEKS, THE ADMINISTRATION WILL RELEASE A HANDBOOK THAT HELPS SCHOOLS AND LOCAL LEADERS IMPLEMENT THE PRECAUTIONS AND STRATEGIES NECESSARY FOR SAFE REOPENING."**

technical support and human resources through the Centers for Disease Control and Prevention (CDC) to help schools implement COVID-19 testing. The Administration will also work to promote access to safe, effective vaccinations for the teachers, school staff and childcare providers who our communities depend on every day.

- **Ensure adequate supplies for school reopening.** To safely reopen, schools need reliable access to supplies like masks and sanitizing products, as well as tests to implement regular COVID-19 screening. As detailed in Goal Four of the National Strategy, the United States will expand the availability of these supplies to meet schools' needs, using the Defense Production Act (DPA) as necessary.

- **Guarantee full access to FEMA disaster relief and emergency assistance for K-12 schools.** The President issues a Presidential Memorandum, *Extend Federal Support to Governors' Use of National Guard to Respond to COVID-19 and to Increase Reimbursement and other Assistance Provided to States*, directing FEMA to authorize and guarantee full access to disaster relief and emergency assistance for K-12 schools under the Stafford Act. This order directs FEMA to fully reimburse states, local governments, territories and tribes for eligible costs. In the coming weeks, FEMA, in consultation with ED and CDC, will work with states and local governments to utilize disaster relief funds to address barriers to school reopening, including purchase of masks and sanitizing products, as well as necessary emergency changes to school ventilation.

- **Support schools in implementing COVID-19 screening testing.** Supporting schools in adopting regular COVID-19 screening testing is a key component of the national strategy to reopen schools while keeping students, teachers, staff, and the surrounding community safe. The federal government will support COVID-19 testing by working with state and local leaders to support the purchase of rapid tests and any necessary expansions in lab capacity, and by providing COVID-19 testing support teams at CDC that help schools develop plans for regular COVID-19 testing, including navigating federal and state requirements, consent, sample collection, and contact tracing. As part of Executive Order *Supporting the Reopening and Continuing Operation of Schools and Early Childhood Education Providers,* the President took action to ensure that COVID-19 tests and other supplies are equitably allocated to support school reopening. The United States will accomplish this by invoking available and appropriate authorities, including the DPA, to purchase and distribute COVID-19 tests and to support states in purchasing COVID-19 tests and testing supplies through purchase guarantees and other means.

> **COVID-19 TESTING SUPPORT TEAMS AT CDC WILL HELP SCHOOLS:**
> - develop plans for regular COVID-19 testing
> - navigate federal and state requirements
> - advise and assist with consent
> - sample collection
> - contact tracing

● **Develop and release detailed technical guidance on safely reopening schools.** School leaders, educators and parents need clear guidance - grounded in science - that they can rely upon to safely re-open and remain open. Executive Order *Supporting the Reopening and Continuing Operation of Schools and Early Childhood Education Providers* directs ED and HHS to develop and release guidance and resources that help schools understand what measures are necessary to support safe reopening, and to continue to provide updated resources as schools' needs and the available evidence evolve. In the coming weeks, ED, in conjunction with CDC, will issue a handbook on school reopening to help answer school administrators' and educators' questions about how to ensure safe operations. The handbook will address topics such as utilizing PPE and other necessary supplies; implementing COVID-19 mitigation measures like physical distancing and cohorting; improving ventilation; increasing staffing; responding to outbreaks; using surge testing and contact tracing to control outbreaks; implementing isolation and quarantine protocols; serving and accommodating students and staff who are immunocompromised or have disabilities/special-needs; and addressing other issues identified by state and local health departments and their education counterparts. The health and safety of children, students, educators, families, and communities is paramount. The Department of Education will work with HHS to ensure that guidance for schools is updated based on the latest science and any developments in the pandemic, including the spread of new coronavirus variants that may have a higher transmission rate. The Administration will always be honest about the challenges we face, directly addressing how and whether changes in the pandemic may impact the reopening of schools or the ability of schools to remain open.

- **Work with governors, local and school leaders, educators and unions to understand barriers and shape policy.** The work to reopen schools is inherently local, and the Administration will be a partner to those on the ground who are steeped in the work of safe reopening. The federal government will convene state and local leaders, educators, labor leaders, and community 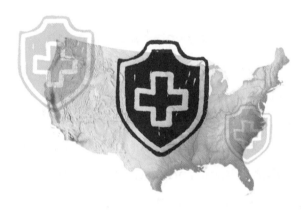 members to collaborate, better understand barriers, and more effectively deploy federal resources to support their efforts. The Administration will work closely to support governors in establishing sound school reopening plans, including assisting them in accessing available federal support through the Department of Education, HHS, and FEMA to accomplish their goals.

- **Create a Safer Schools and Campuses Best Practices Clearinghouse.** To date, states, local jurisdictions and schools have been left on their own to determine how to protect educators, staff, and students; however, even with extremely limited federal support several school districts have taken meaningful steps during the pandemic that can serve as an example to lift up their peers. Executive Order *Supporting the Reopening and Continuing Operation of Schools and Early Childhood Education Providers* directs the creation of a Safer Schools and Campuses Best Practices Clearinghouse to ensure schools and institutions of higher education have access to these types of lessons learned and best practices from other schools and states that have successfully maintained safe operations during the pandemic. These examples will be especially helpful as more federal funding becomes available and districts have the necessary resources to implement effective strategies.

● **Track progress toward school reopening and use of federal funds.** A lack of data on the status of school openings and closures nationwide has left policy makers and the public shockingly in the dark about the true impact of school closures and their effects on low-income students and students of color in particular. Going forward, the federal government will collect and share data on school, district, and state progress toward safely reopening, and will identify opportunities to address challenges — particularly those related to educational equity.

● **Support learning - no matter the setting.** The evidence is clear that getting kids back into school is the best option for children, families, our society and our economy. But some students and educators will not be able to return safely - either because of dangerous COVID-19 rates in their communities, or individual and family health issues. The federal government will continue to prioritize learning for those who cannot be in-person even while working to safely reopen schools. As a first step, the Department of Education will issue guidance to schools on how to best conduct distance learning and how to address the learning loss that occurred over the last several months. President Biden will continue to work with Congress to ensure that schools and districts have adequate funding to provide quality distance learning, including technology, tech support, broadband access, additional staffing, and other supports to students learning both remotely and in person. Additionally, the President's Executive Order *Supporting the Reopening and Continuing Operation of Schools and Early Childhood Education Providers* encourages the Federal Communications Commission to increase connectivity options for students lacking reliable home broadband, so that they can continue to learn if their schools are operating remotely.

Support safe operations at child care centers and at-home providers. With enrollments down and costs up due to COVID-19 precautions, child care providers are struggling to stay afloat while providing vital services to their communities. Due to increased costs and lower enrollment, a recent survey of child care providers showed that most child care providers expect that they will close within a few months without relief, or are uncertain how long they can stay open.[2] If not addressed, child care providers will close and millions of parents will be left to make devastating choices between caring for their children and working to put food on the table. President Biden has called on Congress to provide $25 billion in emergency stabilization to support hard-hit child care providers through the pandemic. These funds would help providers pay rent, utilities, and payroll, as well as cover pandemic-related costs like personal protective equipment, ventilation supplies, smaller group sizes, and alterations to physical spaces that improve safety. The President has also called on Congress to provide $15 billion to help families struggling to afford child care.

● **Provide funding for PPE and other critical supplies through FEMA disaster relief.** In a Presidential Memorandum *Extend Federal Support to Governors' Use of National Guard to Respond to COVID-19 and to Increase Reimbursement and other Assistance Provided to States*, President Biden directed FEMA to reimburse states and local governments for eligible expenses incurred providing PPE emergency relief to child care providers.

● **Update guidance to reflect the reality of child care.** A child care provider can be anything from a large child care center to an individual working in their own home. Providers need guidance that accommodates their circumstances. CDC, in consultation with the HHS Administration for Children and Families, will conduct outreach to child care providers and organizations representing them to assess the need for updates and revisions to guidance to make sure child care providers know what they need to do to reduce the risk and keep themselves, children, families, and staff safe.

---

[2] https://www.naeyc.org/sites/default/files/globally-shared/downloads/PDFs/our-work/public-policy-advocacy/naeyc_policy_crisis_coronavirus_december_survey_data.pdf

- **Provide resources that meet child care providers where they are.** Smaller child care providers and individuals may not have staff or other capacity to help them wade through complex guidance. The Administration will provide simple, at-a-glance resources to help child care providers know what they need to do to address key topics like PPE, ventilation, food preparation, and handling positive cases in their environment.

Support equitable reopening in higher education. College enrollment for high school graduates was down more than 20% in 2020 compared to 2019, and students from low-income families were nearly twice as likely to report canceling their plans to attend college Reopening and keeping colleges open is critical to ensuring that all Americans have a shot at a college credential — but it must be done safely, to protect the health of students, faculty, staff, and the broader community. To support colleges through the pandemic, President Biden has requested that Congress provide an additional $35 billion in emergency stabilization funds for higher education.

- **Support regular COVID-19 testing for under-resourced colleges and universities.** While some universities have successfully implemented regular testing as a means of operating safely during the pandemic, other colleges do not have the resources to do so. The United States will work with states to use federal authorities like the DPA and available state and federal funds to ensure that under-resourced colleges - including community colleges, historically black colleges and universities (HBCUs), Tribal Colleges and minority serving institutions - have access to COVID-19 tests to support reopening.

- **Provide clear guidance on safe college operations.** Given the diversity of settings in which colleges operate and the diversity of services they offer, postsecondary institutions need detailed guidance on recommended COVID-19 protocols that covers a variety of scenarios. The Department of Education, in consultation with the CDC, will conduct outreach to postsecondary institutions and review existing guidance to provide updates that give colleges and universities the latest, science-backed and data-driven recommendations on how and when to open.

- **Work with colleges and universities to conduct outreach to students and staff on vaccination.** With more than 4,000 colleges in the United States representing about 20 million students, colleges and universities are natural

EXECUTIVE ORDER ISSUED

The President issued Executive Order *Protecting Worker Health and Safety* which directs the Occupational Safety and Health Administration (OSHA) to issue updated guidance on COVID-19 worker protections, and to consider whether emergency temporary standards, including with respect to mask wearing, are necessary.

partners for the United States in the effort to get the vaccine to all Americans. The federal government will work with colleges and universities to increase vaccine awareness, reduce hesitancy, and ensure that students, faculty and staff know when they are eligible to get the vaccine, and where to get it. If well-informed by their institutions, college students engaged in remote learning from home may also serve as trusted messengers on vaccine education for their families and communities.

Protect workers and issue stronger worker safety guidance. It is critical that the federal government protect the health and safety of America's workers and take swift action to protect workers from exposure to COVID-19 in the workplace. Millions of Americans, many of whom are people of color, immigrants, and low-wage workers, continue to put their lives on the line to keep the country functioning through the pandemic. They should not have to wonder whether they will make it home from work safely, or whether they will bring the virus to their loved ones or their communities.

The President issued Executive Order *Protecting Worker Health and Safety* which directs the Occupational Safety and Health Administration (OSHA) to issue updated guidance on COVID-19 worker protections, and to consider whether emergency temporary standards, including with respect to mask wearing, are necessary. The President has also called on Congress to authorize OSHA to issue a COVID-19 Protection Standard that covers a broader set of workers, including public sector employees, to provide additional funding for organizations that help keep vulnerable workers safe from COVID-19, and to extend and expand emergency paid leave requirements. The United States will also work to bolster enforcement of health and safety protections.

🛡 **Issue guidance regarding worker safety.** Executive Order *Protecting Worker Health and Safety* directs OSHA, in consultation with CDC, to issue updated guidance on COVID-19 worker protections. This

guidance will be released in the coming weeks and provide a foundation
for businesses to understand how to keep their workplaces safe.

- **Assess the Need for Emergency Temporary Standards.** Executive Order *Protecting Worker Health and Safety* also directs OSHA to immediately start work to determine whether to issue emergency temporary standards, which would create enforceable requirements to protect workers. If issued, this standard would direct employers to adopt plans to keep workers safe and healthy, and make clear how those standards are enforced by OSHA.

- **Strengthen enforcement efforts to protect worker health and safety.** Enforcement is critical to ensuring that employers follow the rules. OSHA will strengthen its enforcement efforts, and it will launch a National Emphasis Program to focus enforcement resources on workplace violations that put the largest number of workers at serious risk. President Biden has also called on Congress to provide additional funds to bolster enforcement efforts.

- **Disseminate guidance to small businesses through the Small Business Administration (SBA).** One key step to ensuring compliance with OSHA guidance is to provide it to businesses as quickly and clearly as possible. SBA will use its touchpoints with businesses - including regional SBA offices and SBA partner networks - to disseminate OSHA guidance widely.

- **Conduct a multilingual outreach campaign to inform workers of their rights.** OSHA will conduct a multilingual outreach campaign to inform workers of their rights, alerting workers that their employer must follow enforceable requirements to protect workers.

- **Support broader availability of PPE, testing, and vaccination for essential workers.** The United States is committed to expanding the availability of PPE for frontline and essential workers. The White House COVID Response team will work with relevant agencies to immediately engage purchases, purchase guarantees, and investments, invoking the DPA as necessary, to ensure the availability of critical PPE and end shortages that have required workers to reuse masks and other protective supplies. Further, by accelerating the pace of vaccinations, the United States will be able to quickly expand vaccine access to frontline and essential workers; the federal government will work with states and localities to ensure that frontline and essential workers have access to the vaccine as quickly as possible. The federal government will also provide support to states for increased public access to COVID-19 testing, from community-based collection locations to options for at-home testing.

- **Provide paid leave to workers that go into quarantine and isolation.** Reliable, robust paid leave is critical to supporting workers to quarantine when exposed to COVID-19 and to isolate when sick. No American should have to choose between putting food on the table and quarantining to prevent further spread of COVID-19. Nearly 1 in 4 workers and close to half of low-income workers lack access to paid sick leave, disproportionately burdening people of color and increasing the risk of COVID-19 infections, hospitalizations, and deaths. Last year, Congress created an emergency paid leave program through the Families First Coronavirus Response Act. The recent coronavirus supplemental package passed by Congress did not extend the emergency paid leave mandate, leaving our country far less prepared to respond to the pandemic. President Biden has called upon Congress to put the requirement back in place and eliminate exemptions so that more workers are covered and expand emergency paid sick and family and

medical leave benefits to over 14 weeks. In the meantime, President Biden will/ has directed his administration to assess whether federal contractors should be required to offer emergency paid leave. The United States will continue to assess other available options to provide payment for quarantine or isolation for workers, teachers, and parents after a positive test in a classroom, place of business, or other situation in which isolation is recommended to prevent the spread of COVID-19.

- **Create conditions for worker vaccination through a national employer pledge.** No worker should have to choose between earning a paycheck and getting the vaccine. The Administration will spearhead a national pledge from businesses to ensure their employees and contractors can take paid time-off to get vaccinated. It will also work with large employers and labor unions to establish on-site vaccination centers, and to provide employees with information about the benefits of vaccination, prioritizing industries and occupations that face heightened risk of COVID-19.

Provide guidance and support to safely open businesses. To maintain safe operations during the pandemic, businesses need to know how to change their practices to protect employees and customers. Many businesses affected by the pandemic—particularly the smallest ones—need additional support to adjust their physical spaces and purchase PPE and other supplies. The United States will immediately work—within the program rules established by Congress—to distribute funds appropriated by the recent COVID-19 relief package to companies hit hardest by COVID-19 and necessary public health restrictions. In addition, President Biden has called on Congress to provide grants to the hardest hit small businesses, and to invest in small business financing programs. Further, the Small Business Administration will work with the Department of Labor to disseminate updated guidance on worker safety and support businesses in implementing it.

> " THE UNITED STATES WILL IMMEDIATELY WORK—WITHIN THE PROGRAM RULES ESTABLISHED BY CONGRESS—TO DISTRIBUTE FUNDS APPROPRIATED BY THE RECENT COVID-19 RELIEF PACKAGE TO COMPANIES HIT HARDEST BY COVID-19 AND NECESSARY PUBLIC HEALTH RESTRICTIONS.

- **Develop and release detailed technical guidance on safely reopening businesses, and provide clear information about the state of the pandemic.** Businesses need to know what they must do to open and operate safely during the pandemic, and they need reliable information on what to expect and how to adapt their operations. The United States will conduct regular, expert-led public briefings on the state of the pandemic and CDC will maintain a public dashboard tracking COVID-19 cases. Provide Further, CDC will continue to develop and update guidance and provide resources for businesses to safely operate.

- **Help small businesses with the costs of operating safely.** The recent COVID-19 supplemental package provided an additional $285 billion for the Paycheck Protection Program to provide loans to small businesses. The United States will, to the extent possible under the law, prioritize these funds for businesses hardest hit by the pandemic. These loans will help small businesses cover the costs of operating safely, including physical changes to the workplace, sanitizing supplies, and PPE.

- **Reduce the costs of pandemic-related supplies.** Persistent shortages have raised the cost of pandemic-related supplies, leaving many business owners footing the bill. The federal government will resolve supply shortages and create steady, reliable demand to drive down prices. Further, the federal government will use its full powers to prevent hoarding and price gouging, including by reviewing and expanding the designated scarce materials under the DPA.

- **Create incentives for safe standards by implementing a safe standards certification program.** Like masking, adhering to the strongest public health protections in the workplace is every American's patriotic duty. When businesses publicly share their commitment to safe standards, it can incentivize other businesses to do the same. The United States will develop a safe standards certification program for businesses, allowing them to self-certify that they are adhering to important public health standards, and providing them with a placard to show their commitment to their communities. The certification standards will align with any forthcoming OSHA guidance, as well as any potential OSHA Emergency Temporary Standard.

Promote Safe Travel. Ensuring that people can safely travel will be critical for families and to jumpstarting the economy, which is why the President issued an executive order that requires mask-wearing on certain public modes of transportation and at ports of entry to the United States. For international air travel, Executive Order *Promoting COVID-19 Safety in Domestic and International Travel* requires a recent negative COVID-19 test result prior to departure and quarantine on arrival, consistent with CDC guidelines. The Executive Order also directs agencies to develop options for expanding public health measures for domestic travel and cross-border land and sea travel and calls for incentives to support and encourage compliance with CDC guidelines on public transportation..

- **Require masking for interstate travel.** Executive Order *Promoting COVID-19 Safety in Domestic and International Travel* requires mask-wearing in airports, on certain modes of public transportation, including many airplanes, trains, maritime vessels, and intercity buses. The Executive Order also directs immediate action to consider additional public health measures in domestic travel.

- **Promote safe international travel.** The United States will implement policies requiring international air travelers to produce a negative COVID-19 test prior to departing for the United States; and to comply with CDC guidelines for self-isolation and self-quarantine upon arrival. The Administration will consult with foreign governments and international organizations regarding the same. The Administration will work with foreign governments and other stakeholders to establish guidelines for and to implement public health measures for safe international travel, including at land and sea borders.

- **Restore FEMA reimbursement for sanitizing public transit.** Public transit is essential for many Americans, and the cost of ensuring that it is safe to use public transportation during the pandemic has been substantial. Local governments' ability to receive support through FEMA disaster relief was rescinded last year, intensifying the budget crunch that state and local governments are experiencing, and threatening the safety of public transit passengers. Through Presidential Memorandum *Extend Federal Support to Governors' Use of National Guard to Respond to COVID-19 and to Increase Reimbursement and other Assistance Provided to States*, President Biden restored funding for these vital sanitation services for states, local governments, tribes and territories.

GOAL SIX

Protect those most at risk and advance equity, including across racial, ethnic and rural/ urban lines

KEY ACTIONS

- Establish the COVID-19 Health Equity Task Force
- Increase data collection and reporting for high risk groups
- Ensure equitable access to critical COVID-19 PPE, tests, therapies, and vaccines
- Expand access to high quality health care
- Expand the clinical and public health workforce, including community-based workers
- Strengthen the social service safety net to address unmet basic needs
- Support communities most at-risk for COVID-19

IMMEDIATE ACTIONS

The President has taken immediate action to implement goal six of the National Strategy by directing immediate steps to identify and address COVID-19 related health inequities and to establish the White House COVID-19 Health Equity Task Force.

- Executive Order: Ensuring an Equitable Pandemic Response and Recovery (January 21, 2021)

The COVID-19 pandemic has exposed and exacerbated severe and pervasive health inequities among communities defined by race, ethnicity, geography, disability, sexual orientation/gender identity and other factors. Addressing this pandemic's devastating toll is both a moral imperative and pragmatic policy.

The Federal Government will address disparities in rates of infection, illness, and death. Specific actions to address equity have been integrated throughout the entirety of the National Strategy for the COVID-19 Response and reflect a whole-of-government approach. This section highlights some, but not all, of the actions described in the National Strategy as well as additional actions that this Administration will take to protect the health of underserved communities and promote resilience in the hardest-hit communities.

In order to prevent COVID-19 illness and death in individuals and communities at greatest risk and advance equity in the federal COVID-19 response, the United States will:

Establish the COVID-19 Health Equity Task Force. The President issued *Executive Order Ensuring an Equitable Pandemic Response and Recovery* which establishes a high-level task force to address COVID-19 related health and social inequities and help coordinate an equitable pandemic response and recovery. The Task Force will convene national experts on health equity and provide specific recommendations to mitigate COVID-19 health inequities.

- **Convene national experts on health equity, including those with lived experience.** The Task Force will be composed of members representing public health, health care, and social service sectors, with maximally diverse backgrounds and perspectives. Additionally, given the whole-of-government approach, federal officials from the Departments of Health and Human Services (HHS), Education, Housing and Urban Development, Agriculture, and Labor will participate.

- **Provide recommendations to mitigate COVID-19 health inequities.** The Task Force will provide timely recommendations to the federal government on how to mitigate health inequities caused or exacerbated by the COVID-19 pandemic and to promote resilience. Such recommendations will focus on the equitable allocation of resources, disbursement of pandemic relief funding and culturally-responsive communication, messaging, and sustained engagement of communities of color and other underserved populations.

Figure 1. COVID-19 has disproportionatetly affected racial and ethnic groups.

Rate ratios compared to White, Non-Hispanic persons

COVID-19 METRIC	AMERICAN INDIANS OR ALASKA NATIVES	ASIAN AMERICANS	BLACKS OR AFRICAN AMERICANS	LATINX
CASES	1.8x	0.6x	1.4x	1.7x
HOSPITALIZATIONS	4.0x	1.2x	3.7x	4.1x
DEATHS	2.6x	1.1x	2.8x	2.8x

Increase data collection and reporting for high risk groups. The fragmented and limited availability of data by race, ethnicity, geography, disability and other demographic variables delays risk recognition and targeted response. Executive Order *Ensuring a Data-Driven Response to COVID-19 and Future High-Consequence Public Health Threats* directs federal agencies to expand their data infrastructure to increase collection and reporting of health data for high risk populations, while reaffirming data privacy. Using these data, the Federal Government will identify high-risk communities, track resource distribution and evaluate the effectiveness of the response. Finally, HHS will optimize data collection from public and private entities to increase the availability of data by race, ethnicity, geography, disability and other sociodemographic variables, as feasible.

- **Expediting and streamlining data collection.** The COVID-19 Health Equity Task Force will develop recommendations for expediting data collection for communities of color and other high-risk groups and identify data sources, proxies, or indices to inform the pandemic response. Further, the Task Force will help to develop a set of recommendations to address data challenges, including data intersectionality, in the longer-term.

- **Identify high-risk communities, track resource distribution and evaluate effectiveness.** The Federal Government will work to stratify all key performance indicators regarding the COVID-19 response by race, ethnicity, geography, disability and other sociodemographic factors to ensure a robust, thoughtful, and equitable response for all communities, including communities of color and other underserved populations. This will include work with CDC to review concerns about vaccine guidelines for people with disabilities and other groups.

- **Increase reporting of federal data.** Centers for Medicare and Medicaid Services (CMS) will work to report Medicare and Medicaid data on COVID-19 testing, cases, vaccinations, hospitalizations, therapeutic utilization, and deaths by race, ethnicity, geography, disability and other sociodemographic factors, as feasible. The Federal Government will work with states to improve the collection and quality of Medicaid data for reporting.

- **Expand data collection for commercially insured populations.** HHS will encourage and support efforts by insurers, pharmacies, labs, state immunization offices and other entities to maximize the availability of data by race, ethnicity, geography, disability and other sociodemographic factors, as feasible.

- **Reaffirm privacy.** We will safeguard privacy, and ensure that these data will be used exclusively for public health services, and that it will not be shared with or used by any federal or state law enforcement activities, including actions by the U.S. Immigration and Customs Enforcement.

Ensure equitable access to critical COVID-19 PPE, tests, therapies, and vaccines. The continued surge of COVID-19 highlights the critical importance of meaningful access to personal protective equipment (PPE), tests, therapies, and vaccines to prevent spread and reduce illness and death in high-risk populations and settings. These resources are acutely needed in many communities, with documented shortages and access barriers across the continuum of care.

As described in Goal Two, the United States will work to ensure that the vaccine is distributed quickly, effectively and equitably, with a focus on making sure that high-risk and hard-to-reach communities are not left behind. We will drive equity in vaccinations by using demographic data to identify hard-hit communities and supporting them, ensuring no out-of-pocket costs for vaccinations, and promoting the distribution of vaccines in those communities. The United States will create as many venues for vaccination as needed, working with state and local entities, in communities and settings that people trust, such as community health centers, rural health clinics and federally run or supported vaccination sites. Engaging with state, local and community-based organizations and trusted health care providers will be central to this effort.

As described in Goal Three, the United States will support COVID-19 screening for schools and other priority populations, ensure that tests are widely available, clarify health insurers' obligation to cover testing, and ensure that testing is free of charge for those who lack health insurance. Regarding therapeutics, the federal government will establish a comprehensive, integrated, and coordinated preclinical drug discovery and development program, with diverse clinical trials, to allow therapeutics to be evaluated and developed rapidly in response to pandemic threats.

As described in Goal Four, the federal government will provide adequate testing and PPE for all medical personnel, first responders, and essential government and private-sector service providers. We will work to replenish depleted supplies in hard-hit, high-risk, and high-need areas and populations, ensuring the affordability and the availability of supplies to key groups including states, schools, workers, health care providers and facilities.

Additional actions include the following:

- **Center equity in the federal response.** The federal government will assess its pandemic response plans and policies to determine whether PPE, tests, vaccines, therapeutics, and other resources have been allocated equitably. Federal agencies will modify plans and policies as necessary, with consideration to the effect of any proposed policy changes on resource distribution and access in the hardest-hit communities. The Task Force will provide recommendations on addressing structural barriers that impede equitable access. We will work with the public and private sectors to accelerate equitable access to resources.

- **Update state pandemic plans.** The Centers for Disease Control and Prevention (CDC) will work with states and localities to update their pandemic plans to describe how they have or will provide equitable access to COVID-19 resources within highly vulnerable communities, including Tribal communities, using CDC's Social Vulnerability Index or other indices as appropriate. HHS will provide additional tools to inform equitable pandemic planning, such as mapping pharmacy deserts across the country, and provide technical assistance as needed.

- 🛡 **Strengthen enforcement of anti-discrimination requirements.** HHS and other federal agencies will provide guidance and increase enforcement regarding non-discrimination requirements in access to and availability of COVID-19 care and treatment. The Task Force will provide recommendations on federal guidance for crisis standards of care.

- 🛡 **Launch a targeted, stakeholder- and data-informed vaccination communication campaign.** Multiple reports and surveys document vaccine hesitancy across populations, reflecting the realities of medical experimentation and other abuses for some people in communities of color. As described in Goal 2, HHS will support a large-scale campaign to promote trust and build vaccine confidence, in close collaboration with doctors and nurses, faith-based, civic, and advocacy groups working with or representing the hardest-hit communities.

- 🛡 **Prioritize diverse and inclusive representation in clinical research.** Federally-sponsored clinical trials for COVID-19 therapeutics, preventatives, and other emerging technologies will require diverse and inclusive representation. The Administration will be asked to monitor and assist recruitment and retention of racial, ethnic and other demographic groups and subgroups into clinical trials to increase population-wide data on safety and effectiveness.

Figure 2.

Racial/Ethnic Distribution of Health Care Workers

TOTAL AND SELECT OCCUPATIONS, 2019

	White	Black	Hispanic	Asian	Other

	ALL HEALTH CARE WORKERS	AIDES AND PERSONAL CARE WORKERS	DIRECT CONTACT SUPPORT WORKERS	HEALTH CARE PROVIDERS
Other	3%	3%	3%	3%
Asian	7%	7%	5%	10%
Hispanic	13%	13%	17%	10%
Black	16%	29%	22%	10%
White	60%	45%	53%	57%

Expand access to high quality health care. The federal government will work to expand affordable coverage to increase access to care during this pandemic, and the Task Force will provide recommendations to align federal incentives with improved clinical outcomes. Specific actions include efforts to increase funding for community health centers, provide greater assistance to safety net institutions, strengthen home- and community-based services, expand mental health care, and support care and research on the effects of long COVID.

- **Increase funding for community health centers.** The nation's 1,400 community health centers provide primary health care to nearly 30 million people—the majority of whom are people of color—in every state and territory, including 1 in 5 rural residents, 1 in 3 living in poverty, and more than 1 million of both agricultural workers and people experiencing homelessness. The Administration has asked Congress to increase funding to expand access to health services for underserved populations.

- **Provide greater assistance to safety net institutions.** CMS will be asked to review the program definitions for safety net providers to ensure that safety net institutions that disproportionately serve marginalized communities are allocated funding and resources equitably.

- **Strengthen support for home and community based services.** The President has proposed significant investments in home and community based services as part of his plan to Build Back Better. HHS, including CMS and the Administration for Community Living, will be asked to identify opportunities and funding mechanisms to provide greater support for individuals receiving home and community based services, with particular attention to people with disabilities and the home care workforce crisis.

- **Support care and research on long-term COVID effects.** For those individuals who contracted the novel coronavirus, HHS will establish a system for monitoring long-term health sequelae and understanding treatment needs, including in people of color.

● **Expand mental health services.** Individuals and communities, including the health workforce, are experiencing emotional trauma and exacerbation of existing mental health and substance use issues during this pandemic, requiring increased availability of behavioral health services. We have asked the Congress for increased funding for the Substance Abuse and Mental Health Services Administration and Health Resources and Services Administration to expand such services, including in medically-underserved communities.

Expand the clinical and public health workforce, including community-based workers. Over the last decade, state and local public health agencies have lost nearly a quarter of their workforce. In order to assure equitable PPE distribution, testing, contact tracing, social support for quarantine and isolation, and vaccination, there must be sufficient workforce to serve the communities in greatest need.

As described in Goal Three, through Executive Order *Improving and Expanding Access to Care and Treatment for COVID-19,* the President has outlined immediate steps to increase clinical capacity by targeted deployment of federal assets, workforce, and facilities to states to bolster critical care capacity in hotspots. *Improving and Expanding Access to Care and Treatment for COVID-19* encourages states and providers to take all available actions to support and expand the health care workforce to address staff shortages, and increases access to programs that meet the long-term health needs of patients recovering from COVID-19 through technical assistance and support to community health centers.

● **Create a United States Public Health Workforce Program of new community based workers to assist with testing, tracing and vaccination.** As described in Goal Three, this program will mobilize at least 100,000 people to conduct culturally-responsive outreach and engagement, testing, contact tracing, and other critical functions. These workers will be recruited from the communities they serve in order to facilitate trusting relationships with local residents. HHS and DOL will explore mechanisms to create and connect workers to "career ladder" programs and consider reimbursement mechanisms to encourage health care institutions and community-based organizations to employ them post-pandemic.

- **Deploy federal officials to under-resourced areas.** The federal government will deploy federal workers to assist with the COVID-19 response in high risk communities as needed. Such workers include officials from HHS' Centers for Disease Control and Prevention, U.S. Public Health Service Commissioned Corps, and National Health Services Corps, as well as officials from the Federal Emergency Management Agency, Veterans Administration, and Department of Agriculture.

Strengthen the social service safety net to address unmet basic needs. With millions of families already struggling pre-pandemic to meet basic needs, including food, housing and transportation, COVID-19 has exacerbated these challenges. These challenges contribute to difficulties by many to adhere to public health guidance regarding social distancing and quarantine/isolation. The Administration is committed to addressing these needs in multiple ways, including providing paid sick leave, child care support and rental assistance, with Congressional appropriations. Additionally, it will undertake agency actions to designate COVID-19 health equity leads and extend flexibilities to select programs during the pandemic, as well support community-based, multi-sector efforts to align health and social interventions.

- **Designate federal agency COVID-19 health equity leads.** Reflecting a whole-of-government approach, the Departments of Health and Human Services, Education, Agriculture, Housing and Urban Development, and Labor each will designate a COVID-19 equity lead, to ensure a coordinated and comprehensive approach to meeting individual and family health and social needs. HHS will regularly convene and coordinate the work of these health equity leads, who may also participate in the COVID-19 Health Equity Task Force at the discretion of the Chair.

- **Extend flexibilities initiated during the pandemic.** The federal government has taken steps to facilitate eligibility determinations and enrollment for individuals in public benefit programs, including by simplifying documentation and reducing in-person interview requirements. We will pursue extending these and other flexibilities throughout the pandemic response and recovery.

- **Facilitate linkages between clinical and social services.** Given the increased need for social services during this pandemic, HHS will identify opportunities and mechanisms to support screening, referral and linkage to social services during COVID-19 testing and vaccination programs, with particular focus on expanding community-based, multisector partnerships that can align health and social interventions.

Figure 3.

Percent of Nonelderly Adults with Selected Health Conditions by Race/Ethnicity, 2018

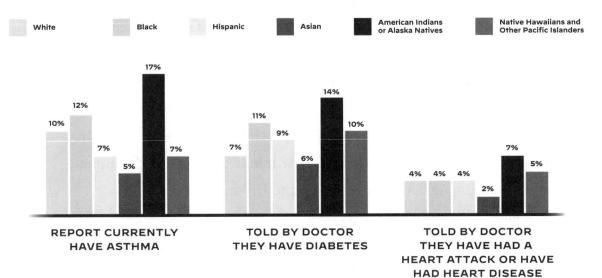

Legend: White | Black | Hispanic | Asian | American Indians or Alaska Natives | Native Hawaiians and Other Pacific Islanders

REPORT CURRENTLY HAVE ASTHMA: 10%, 12%, 7%, 5%, 17%, 7%

TOLD BY DOCTOR THEY HAVE DIABETES: 7%, 11%, 9%, 6%, 14%, 10%

TOLD BY DOCTOR THEY HAVE HAD A HEART ATTACK OR HAVE HAD HEART DISEASE: 4%, 4%, 4%, 2%, 7%, 5%

Support communities most at-risk for COVID-19. The Administration is committed to supporting populations that are most vulnerable to COVID-19. Whether residing in congregate settings, serving as essential workers, having disabilities or bearing the burden of chronic medical conditions, these most vulnerable populations are disproportionately made up of people of color. The Federal Government will take steps to ensure these populations have access to adequate PPE and the resources to implement appropriate testing and vaccination strategies. The CDC will develop and update clear public health guidance for such high-risk institutions and settings to further minimize the risk of COVID infection. Additionally, the following policies will be implemented to address particular high-risk communities:

- **Ensure the Federal Bureau of Prisons and U.S. Immigration and Customs Enforcement (ICE) detention facilities are following sound public health guidance.** The President will issue an Executive Order to require the Bureau of Prisons and ICE detention facilities to evaluate their COVID-19 protocols, release data on the spread of COVID-19 in facilities, and use federal grant programs to create incentives for state and local facilities to adhere to sound public health guidance.

- **Supporting nursing home and long-term care facility residents and staff.** HHS and the Center for Medicare and Medicaid Services will strengthen Long Term Care facility guidance, funding, and requirements around infection control policies; support Long Term Care staffing levels sufficient to ensure patient safety, and support the accelerated distribution of vaccines to residential care settings.

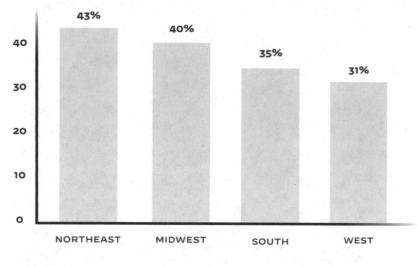

Share of Total COVID-19 Deaths that Occured in Long-term Care Facilities

SOURCE: COVID Tracking Project

COMMUNITIES MOST AT-RISK FOR COVID-19

As the pandemic has progressed, a clearer understanding has developed for the communities most at risk for severe COVID-19 disease and for infection in general. Review of those same risk factors also helps elucidate some of the mechanisms that—in addition to structural inequality and systemic racism—help to drive COVID-19 inequities by race and ethnicity. According to the CDC, several groups have higher-risk for COVID-19 infection, illness or death. Among these are older adults, those with chronic medical conditions, rural communities, and individuals living or working in congregate settings.

Older adults. Compared to younger adults, older adults are more likely to require hospitalization if they get COVID-19. Throughout the pandemic, nearly 8 of 10 COVID-19 deaths in the United States have been in adults ages 65 and older.

Refugees to the United States, especially those who are recently resettled, may experience living arrangements or working conditions that put them at greater risk of getting COVID-19. Some refugees also have limited access to health care, as well as certain underlying medical conditions that put them at increased risk of severe illness from COVID-19, compared to the rest of the U.S. population.

Adults with chronic medical conditions. Adults of any age with certain underlying medical conditions are at increased risk for severe COVID-19. Conditions associated with increased risk of severe COVID-19 include: cancer, chronic kidney disease, chronic obstructive pulmonary disease (COPD), Down Syndrome, heart disease, immunocompromised state from solid organ transplant, obesity, pregnancy, sickle cell disease, smoking and type 2 diabetes mellitus. Of note, differential prevalence of disease by race and ethnicity for many of these conditions contributes to the greater risk for severe COVID-19 in communities of color. Black Americans, for example, experience higher rates of the majority of these conditions.

Rural communities. In general, rural Americans tend to have higher rates of cigarette smoking, high blood pressure, and obesity as well as less access to health care which can negatively affect health outcomes. They are also less likely to have health insurance. The combination of factors portends a higher risk of severe COVID-19 among those who contract the disease.

Congregate settings. Congregate settings are defined as environments where a number of people reside, meet or gather in close proximity for either a limited or extended period of time. Examples include homeless shelters, correctional and detention facilities, nursing homes and long-term care facilities, refugee communities, and group homes.

- **Homeless services** are often provided in congregate settings, which could facilitate the spread of infection. Because many people who are homeless are older adults or have underlying medical conditions, they may also be at increased risk for severe illness.

- People in **correctional and detention facilities** are at greater risk for some illnesses, such as COVID-19, because of close living arrangements with other people.

- The communal nature of **nursing homes and long-term care facilities**, and the population served (generally older adults often with underlying medical conditions), put those living in nursing homes at increased risk of infection and severe illness from COVID-19.

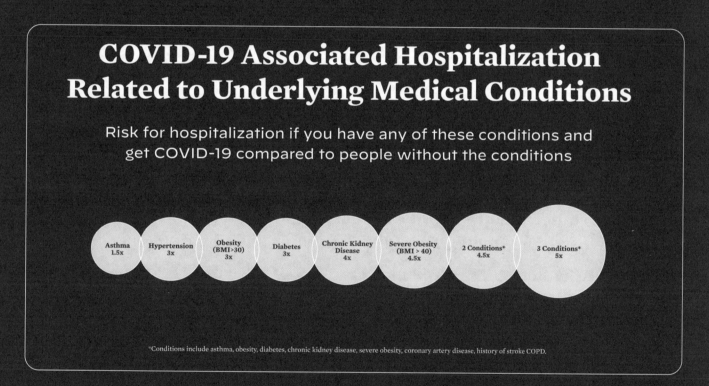

COVID-19 Associated Hospitalization Related to Underlying Medical Conditions

Risk for hospitalization if you have any of these conditions and get COVID-19 compared to people without the conditions

| Asthma 1.5x | Hypertension 3x | Obesity (BMI>30) 3x | Diabetes 3x | Chronic Kidney Disease 4x | Severe Obesity (BMI > 40) 4.5x | 2 Conditions* 4.5x | 3 Conditions* 5x |

*Conditions include asthma, obesity, diabetes, chronic kidney disease, severe obesity, coronary artery disease, history of stroke COPD.

Individuals with disabilities, including those who live in group homes and those receiving home- and community-based services. In both settings, several factors may facilitate the introduction and spread of COVID-19. Some of these factors include residents employed outside the home, residents who require close contact with staff or Direct Service Providers, residents who have trouble understanding information or practicing preventive measures, and residents in shared living spaces.

Agricultural industry workers, including meat packers and migrant farm workers, where employees live and/or work in close proximity and faced severe outbreaks.

Restore U.S. leadership globally and build better preparedness for future threats

KEY ACTIONS

— Restore the U.S. relationship with the World Health Organization and seek to strengthen and reform it
— Surge the international public health & humanitarian response
— Restore U.S. leadership to the international COVID-19 response and advance global health security and diplomacy
— Build better biopreparedness and expand resilience for biological threats

IMMEDIATE ACTIONS

The President has taken immediate action to implement goal seven of the National Strategy by directing actions to re-engage with and seek to strengthen and reform the World Health Organization (WHO), restore a strong U.S. role in the global COVID-19 response, and advance global health security and international institutions to prevent, detect, and respond to future biological catastrophes.

— Presidential Letters: Re-engage with the WHO (January 20, 2021)
— U.S Global Leadership to Strengthen the Global COVID-19 Response, Global Health Security, and Biological Preparedness (January 21, 2021)

America's withdrawal from the international arena has impeded progress on a global COVID-19 response and left the United States more vulnerable to future pandemics. U.S. international engagement to combat COVID-19, promote health, and advance global health security will save lives, promote economic recovery, and build better resilience against future biological catastrophes.

In a matter of months, COVID-19 has infected [over 90 million people worldwide, has caused over 2 million deaths], and has erased decades of gains in global health and development. For the first time since 1998, global poverty is increasing. Nowhere will the effects of this pandemic be more devastating than on the world's most vulnerable communities. The pandemic is reversing hard-fought gains in global health, including routine immunizations, maternal and child health, and the fight against tuberculosis, malaria, and HIV/AIDS, and is increasing the risk of gender-based violence. The pandemic has also disproportionately affected women and girls and significantly deepened existing gender inequalities around the world. At the same time, it will be impossible to plug urgent holes in the leaky global pandemic supply chain, outdated biological early warning and alert system, and weak public health infrastructure unless we simultaneously lay the foundation for the system we need for a better future. COVID-19 outbreaks are likely to occur in the United States and globally for years, even after the introduction of a safe and effective vaccine. While the federal government will immediately fight COVID-19, it must also be prepared for another biological threat — whether naturally-occurring, deliberate, or accidental — to arrive.

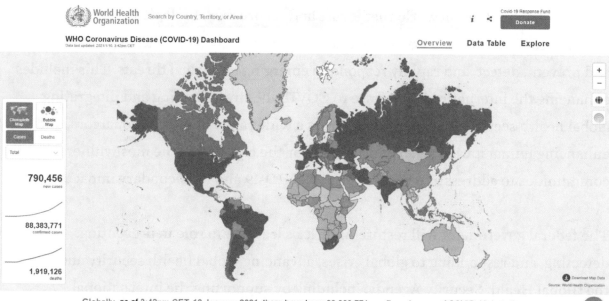

Globally, as of 3:42pm CET, 10 January 2021, there have been 88,383,771 confirmed cases of COVID-19, including 1,919,126 deaths, reported to WHO.

Cumulative COVID-19 Deaths per 100,000 Population

January 2021

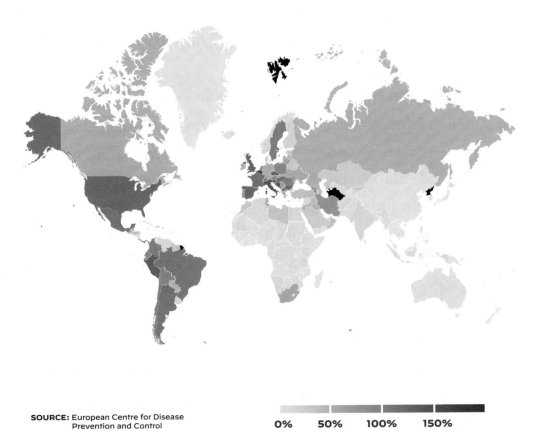

SOURCE: European Centre for Disease Prevention and Control

0%　50%　100%　150%

Epidemic and pandemic preparedness, health security, and global health are essential elements of U.S. foreign policy, national security affairs, humanitarian response, and development policy. Recognizing that COVID-19 is a global challenge that requires a global response, the United States will work with other countries to combat COVID-19 and achieve a world that is safe and secure from biological catastrophes. The United States will engage diplomatically to fight COVID-19 and to prepare for and prevent, detect, and rapidly respond to emerging biological threats. This includes enhancing the international response to COVID-19, strengthening and integrating global health security considerations across a wide range of international fora, and enhancing humanitarian relief and support for the capacity of the most vulnerable communities to address and recover from COVID-19 and its secondary impacts.

The federal government will restore America's leadership role in preventing, detecting, and responding to global crises, advancing global health security and the Global Health Security Agenda, including by supporting the international pandemic response effort, providing humanitarian relief and global health assistance, and building resilience for future epidemics and pandemics. The United States will immediately re-engage with partners to effectively combat COVID-19, show effective leadership in the global COVID-19 response, and work to prevent emerging and future biological events from creating further U.S. and global human and economic catastrophe. The federal government will direct urgent actions in the near term, while also laying the groundwork to build biopreparedness, establish a resilient global health security system, and strengthen global health.

Restore the U.S. relationship with the World Health Organization and seek to strengthen it. The World Health Organization (WHO) plays a critical role in coordinating the international response to COVID-19 and improving the health of all people. It is essential that the United States government participate in the WHO and work to strengthen and reform the organization. On May 29, 2020, the prior Administration sent formal notification to the WHO of its intent to withdraw from the organization, effective July 6, 2021, one year after notification as outlined by the U.S. ratification to the WHO Constitution. This move has not only alienated international partners and jeopardized global health and development gains, it has also made it more difficult for the United States to participate in strengthening the international health security architecture - including the WHO - required for its own national security.

On his first day in office, President Biden sent letters informing the UN Secretary-General and the WHO Director General of his decision to cease the previous Administration's process of withdrawing from the WHO. The United States will participate in the WHO Executive Board meeting in January, and will seek action to strengthen and reform the WHO.

- **Re-engage with the WHO, including to control COVID-19.** On January 20, the President sent letters to the UN Secretary-General and the WHO Director General stating that the United States will remain a member of the WHO and meet its financial obligations.

- **Participate in the WHO Executive Board.** On January 21, Chief Medical Advisor and NIAID Director, Dr. Anthony Fauci will deliver a message from President Biden to the WHO Executive Board to restore U.S. leadership and scientific credibility back to our work with the organization.

- **Seek to strengthen and reform the WHO.** In 2021, the United States will work with the WHO and its Member States on an agenda to strengthen and reform the organization so that it can effectively achieve its goal of improving health for all people and markedly improve global health security.

Surge the international COVID-19 public health & humanitarian response. COVID-19 has highlighted weaknesses in public health capacity in the United States and around the world, as well as the lack of available international institutions to foster rapid action to control disease and save lives during a biological crisis. The need for functional global outbreak response has never been more clear. Multilateral leadership and effective communication are vital to coordinate an effective response to mitigate the consequences of diseases—both COVID-19 and future threats to come—and ultimately save lives.

At the same time, the COVID-19 pandemic is reversing hard-won gains in childhood vaccination coverage, fighting tuberculosis, HIV, malaria, malnutrition, maternal and child mortality, sexual and reproductive health and rights, poverty and so much more. An ambitious global posture in fighting and recovering from the COVID-19 pandemic presents the United States with an opportunity to restore its global health leadership, reset and drive action to advance the Sustainable Development Goals, make gains toward achieving Universal Health Coverage, and build a stronger global foundation for preventing, detecting, and responding to future biological threats.

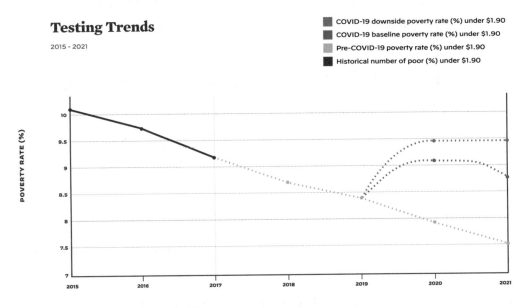

Testing Trends

2015 - 2021

- COVID-19 downside poverty rate (%) under $1.90
- COVID-19 baseline poverty rate (%) under $1.90
- Pre-COVID-19 poverty rate (%) under $1.90
- Historical number of poor (%) under $1.90

Source: Poverty and Shared Prosperity 2020, PoycalNet

The United States will commit to multilateralism in the international COVID-19 public health and humanitarian response. The President will restore U.S. leadership on global COVID-19 response and health security, laying out an active role for the United States in surging the health and humanitarian response to COVID-19, and supporting global vaccine distribution and research and development for treatments, tests, and vaccines. The United States will support the Access to COVID-19 Tools (ACT) Accelerator and join the COVID-19 Vaccines Global Access (COVAX) Facility and seek to strengthen other existing multilateral initiatives, such as the Coalition for Epidemic Preparedness Innovations; Gavi, the Vaccine Alliance; and the Global Fund to Fight AIDS, tuberculosis, and malaria. The United States will also take steps to enhance humanitarian relief and support for the capacity of the most vulnerable communities to prevent, detect, respond to, mitigate, and recover from impacts of COVID-19, such as food insecurity and malnutrition, gender-based violence, and economic devastation. The federal government will restore U.S. leadership to the global COVID-19 public health and humanitarian response and mitigate secondary impacts. The federal government will:

- **Join COVAX and support multilateral cooperation on COVID-19 research and development, vaccination, diagnostics, and therapeutics.** The United States will join the approximately 190 other countries that participate in the global vaccine distribution arrangement (COVAX), engage with the COVID-19 Tools (ACT) accelerator, and make recommendations on a framework for donating future U.S. vaccine surplus. The Biden-Harris Administration will seek funding from Congress to strengthen and sustain these efforts, as well as other existing multilateral initiatives involved in fighting COVID-19, such as the Coalition for Epidemic Preparedness Innovations; Gavi, the Vaccine Alliance; and the Global Fund to Fight AIDS, TB and Malaria.

- **Strengthen the humanitarian response.** The United States will work to support international humanitarian relief and resilience efforts aimed to mitigate the impacts of COVID-19 and to support the capacity of most vulnerable communities to prevent, respond to, and mitigate primary and secondary impacts of COVID-19. The Administration will engage women and other vulnerable groups as part of these efforts.

- **Secure funding for the global response.** The Administration will seek resources and empower State, USAID, CDC, the U.S. International Development Finance Corporation, the Millenium Challenge Corporation, and Treasury to effectively allocate those resources to respond to COVID-19 and address its secondary impacts, including global health, food insecurity, increasing rates of gender-based violence, women's health, the education crisis, and other needs.

- **Develop an international biological and response framework.** The Administration is committed to establishing an international biological and response framework across the U.S. government that clarifies roles, prioritizes actions, and identifies existing gaps in our response to emerging global high-consequence infectious disease threats, establishes standard operating procedures between USAID and CDC, and ensures readiness of deployable rapid response capabilities.

- **Mitigate secondary impacts of COVID-19 on health and development and restore U.S. leadership in global health, humanitarian and development organizations, and international financial institutions.** The federal government will mitigate the secondary impacts of COVID-19 and strengthen bilateral U.S. programs in HIV, TB, malaria, and other health systems strengthening efforts; seek to advance global debt relief efforts; work to improve health outcomes for women and girls, including through recommitting to sexual and reproductive health and rights and maternal and child health and nutrition programs; and advance gender parity, diversity, and inclusion.

Restore U.S. leadership to the international COVID-19 response and advance global health security and diplomacy. Naturally occurring, accidental, or deliberate biological events— whether potentially catastrophic like a pandemic or smaller scale like an emerging Ebola outbreak or targeted anthrax attack— pose immense threats to national and international security. Meanwhile, the risk of catastrophic biological events is growing, sparked by our interconnected world, risk of zoonotic spillover, advances in technologies like gene editing and DNA synthesis without adequate norms and oversight, and vulnerabilities in global preparedness and resilience laid bare by COVID-19.

The COVID-19 pandemic highlights the importance of—as well as existing limitations in—international institutions and governance for infectious disease prevention and control, the necessity of accurate understandings of domestic preparedness and resilience, and the critical need for early, capable national leadership to coordinate an effective response. In 2014, the Obama-Biden Administration launched the Global Health Security Agenda, a multilateral effort to advance epidemic preparedness, in collaboration with countries and international organizations around the world, designed to raise political salience, marshal resources, and coordinate measured action to prevent, detect and respond to biological threats.

The federal government will immediately re-engage with its global partners, including through multilateral mechanisms, to control the COVID-19 pandemic and to build the public health cooperation and institutions we need to prevent, detect, and respond to future biological catastrophes. The United States will promote sustainable global health and global health security, rebuild health security alliances, elevate U.S. efforts to support the Global Health Security Agenda, and revitalize U.S. leadership.

The United States will advance global health security financing, seek to harmonize crisis response and early warning systems for public health emergencies, and strengthen global pandemic supply chains. The United States will also work within the UN Security Council and with partner countries to strengthen multilateral public health and humanitarian cooperation on the COVID-19 response, global institutions to combat disease, and a global health security architecture to prevent, detect, and respond to future epidemic and pandemic threats. The federal government will:

- **Restore White House and diplomatic leadership on COVID-19 and emerging biological threats.** The Biden-Harris Administration will reinstate White House leadership on global health security, including by reinstating the National Security Council Directorate on Global Health Security and Biodefense. The Administration will also designate senior leaders to provide leadership across departments and agencies for the global COVID-19 response and to advance global health and health security diplomacy.

- **Commit to multilateralism.** The United States will work with partners, including the G-7, G-20, the UN, African Union, ASEAN, and other partners to support the global response to and recovery from the pandemic. This will include working with international partners, the WHO and the broader UN system, including the United Nations Security Council, to support a more collective and robust multilateral response on COVID-19 and global health security. The Administration will promote stronger global governance of global health and epidemic preparedness, act on the UN Secretary-General's call to put women and girls at the center of global recovery efforts, and signal U.S. leadership and interest in coordinating in the international response and on multilateral vaccine and supply chain initiatives.

- **Commit to building sustainable health security architecture.** The United States will advance health security country capacity and global institutions to mitigate biological catastrophes. The United States will also seek to explore the establishment of a new position in the office of the UN Secretary-General of a facilitator for high-consequence biological threats, particularly for events involving significant collaboration and equities across the United Nations. The Administration will prepare specific U.S. commitments to advance new mechanisms for health security financing, establish sustainable health security financing, implement multilateral vaccine development and distribution, secure global and regional pandemic supply chains, and build a stronger international health emergency early warning system that is biased toward rapid, transparent, and coordinated global action when new epidemic and pandemic threats emerge.

- **Make and execute commitments to mitigate future biological catastrophes,** including by:
    - Developing stronger institutions focused on harmonizing crisis response for emerging public health emergencies;
    - Supporting the establishment of a mechanism to sustainably finance health security capacity;
    - Strengthening the International Health Regulations, working with partners and international organizations;
    - Reducing racial and ethnic disparities in COVID-19 global response and disproportionate impacts on marginalized and indigenous communities, women and girls, and other groups;
    - Reviewing and developing priorities for multilateral fora geared at reducing deliberate and accidental biological risks; and
    - Fighting climate change as a driver of health threats.

Build better biopreparedness and expand resilience for biological threats. Biological risks are increasing and accelerating due to a variety of trends, including zoonotic diseases that spill over to humans; a changing climate; and advances in technology that make it easier, cheaper and faster to make and modify dangerous agents. In addition, COVID-19 outbreaks are likely to occur in the United States and globally for years even after the introduction of a safe and effective vaccine. During the Biden-Harris Administration, it is likely that other biological events - including the potential for another high consequence or pandemic event - will occur. The United States must strengthen its capacity to swiftly counter potentially catastrophic biological events.

The Biden-Harris Administration is committed to strengthening biopreparedness and the capacity to counter COVID-19 and future biological threats. On January 20, President Biden restored the White House National Security Council Directorate for Global Health Security and Biodefense established by the Obama-Biden Administration. On January 21, he issued a National Security Directive directing steps to improve long-term biopreparedness in the United States.

The federal government will reconstitute a White House and Administration-wide infrastructure for monitoring and responding to emerging biological risks. And to improve the United States' preparedness, the Administration will work to secure funding and Congressional support to establish an integrated, National Center for Epidemic Forecasting and Outbreak Analytics to modernize global early warning and trigger systems to prevent, detect, and respond to biological threats. The United States will also review and seek to strengthen our pandemic supply chain, public health workforce, medical countermeasure development and distribution, bioeconomic investment and technology related risks, and vital other elements of U.S. biodefense.

The Biden-Harris Administration will take immediate action to improve the national COVID-19 response, while simultaneously building better biopreparedness in the United States for future biological events, including re-emerging outbreaks of COVID-19. These include actions to:

- **Advance epidemic and pandemic preparedness in the United States for COVID-19 and future public health emergencies.** President Biden issued a National Security Directive, initiating a review of U.S. policy on emerging domestic and global biological risks and national biopreparedness policies and then addresses any outstanding issues, including work to expand the pandemic supply chain, workforce, hospital preparedness, countermeasure development and distribution, epidemic forecasting and modeling, pathogen-tracking, bio-related intelligence, bioeconomic investment, and strengthening preparedness for bio events.

- **Monitor current and emerging biological threats** to provide early warning for decision-makers as biological risks emerge so that leaders can take urgent action to detect, track, and control disease outbreaks before they become catastrophic.

- **Secure funding to build back better U.S. biopreparedness,** including bolstering national testing supply and laboratory capacity; vaccine and therapeutic research, development, distribution, and dispensing; hospital preparedness; the community and public health workforce; the U.S. pandemic supply chain and Strategic National Stockpile, and other vital capabilities to build preparedness against COVID-19 and future biological catastrophes.

- **Establish a National Center for Epidemic Forecasting and Outbreak Analytics.** The United States will modernize data systems and establish global early warning and trigger systems to prevent, detect, and respond to emerging biological threats.

- **Develop sustainable U.S. infrastructure for biological and pandemic events,** including but not limited to:
  - Strengthening State, local, tribal, and territorial public health infrastructure and personnel;
  - Improving data integration and information technology systems at the local, state and federal level;
  - Developing a framework of pandemic readiness with specific action triggers for large-scale biological events;
  - Revitalizing the Strategic National Stockpile;
  - Building long-term U.S. hospital preparedness;

- Security the pandemic supply chain;
- Growing the community and public health workforce;
- Building preparedness for emerging biotechnology risks while investing in the bioeconomy;
- Deterring and defending against deliberate biological attacks;
- Countering antimicrobial resistance; and
- Mitigating the health security impacts of climate change.

EXECUTIVE ORDER

ORGANIZING AND MOBILIZING THE UNITED STATES GOVERNMENT TO PROVIDE A UNIFIED AND EFFECTIVE RESPONSE TO COMBAT COVID19 AND TO PROVIDE UNITED STATES LEADERSHIP ON GLOBAL HEALTH AND SECURITY

By the authority vested in me as President by the Constitution and the laws of the United States of America, it is hereby ordered as follows:

Section 1. Purpose. The Federal Government must act swiftly and aggressively to combat coronavirus disease 2019 (COVID-19). To that end, this order creates the position of Coordinator of the COVID-19 Response and Counselor to the President and takes other steps to organize the White House and activities of the Federal Government to combat COVID-19 and prepare for future biological and pandemic threats.

Sec. 2. Organizing the White House to Combat COVID-19. (a) In order to effectively, fully, and immediately respond to COVID-19, there is established within the Executive Office of the President the position of Coordinator of the COVID-19 Response and Counselor to the President (COVID-19 Response Coordinator) and the position of Deputy Coordinator of the COVID-19 Response. The COVID-19 Response Coordinator shall report directly to the President; advise and assist the President and executive departments and agencies (agencies) in responding to the COVID-19 pandemic; coordinate all elements of the COVID-19 response; and perform such duties as the President may otherwise direct. These duties shall include:

(i) coordinating a Government-wide effort to reduce disparities in the response, care, and treatment of COVID-19, including racial and ethnic disparities;

(ii) coordinating the Federal Government's efforts to produce, supply, and distribute personal protective equipment, vaccines, tests, and other supplies for the Nation's COVID-19 response, including through the use of the Defense Production Act, as amended (50 U.S.C. 4501 et seq.);

(iii) coordinating the Federal Government's efforts to expand COVID-19 testing and the use of testing as an effective public health response;

(iv) coordinating the Federal Government's efforts to support the timely, safe, and effective delivery of COVID-19 vaccines to the United States population;

(v) coordinating the Federal Government's efforts to support the safe reopening and operation of schools, child care providers, and Head Start programs, and to help ensure the continuity of educational and other services for young children and elementary and secondary students during the COVID-19 pandemic; and

(vi) coordinating, as appropriate, with State, local, Tribal, and territorial authorities.

(b) The COVID-19 Response Coordinator shall have the authority to convene principals from relevant agencies, in consultation with the Assistant to the President for Domestic Policy (APDP) on matters involving the domestic COVID-19 response, and in consultation with the Assistant to the President for National Security Affairs (APNSA) on matters involving the global COVID-19 response. The COVID-19 Response Coordinator shall also coordinate any corresponding deputies and interagency processes.

(c) The COVID-19 Response Coordinator may act through designees in performing these or any other duties.

Sec. 3. United States Leadership on Global Health and Security and the Global COVID-19 Response.

(a) Preparing to Respond to Biological Threats and Pandemics. To identify, monitor, prepare for, and, if necessary, respond to emerging biological and pandemic threats:

(i) The APNSA shall convene the National Security Council (NSC) Principals

Committee as necessary to coordinate the Federal Government's efforts to address such threats and to advise the President on the global response to and recovery from COVID-19, including matters regarding: the intersection of the COVID-19 response and other national security equities; global health security; engaging with and strengthening the World Health Organization; public health, access to healthcare, and the secondary impacts of COVID-19; and emerging biological risks and threats, whether naturally occurring, deliberate, or accidental.

(ii) Within 180 days of the date of this order, the APNSA shall, in coordination with relevant agencies, the COVID-19 Response Coordinator, and the APDP, complete a review of and recommend actions to the President concerning emerging domestic and global biological risks and national biopreparedness policies. The review and recommended actions shall incorporate lessons from the COVID-19 pandemic and, among other things, address: the readiness of the pandemic supply chain, healthcare workforce, and hospitals; the development of a framework of pandemic readiness with specific triggers for when agencies should take action in response to large-scale biological events; pandemic border readiness; the development and distribution of medical countermeasures; epidemic forecasting and modeling; public health data modernization; bio-related intelligence; bioeconomic investments; biotechnology risks; the development of a framework for coordinating with and distributing responsibilities as between the Federal Government and State, local, Tribal, and territorial authorities; and State, local, Tribal, and territorial preparedness for biological events.

(b) NSC Directorate on Global Health Security and Biodefense. There shall be an NSC Directorate on Global Health Security and Biodefense, which shall be headed by a Senior Director for Global Health Security and Biodefense. The Senior Director shall be responsible for monitoring current and emerging biological threats, and shall report concurrently to the APNSA and to the COVID-19 Response Coordinator on matters relating to COVID-19. The Senior Director shall oversee the Global Health Security Agenda Interagency Review Council, which was established pursuant to Executive Order 13747 of November 4, 2016 (Advancing the Global Health Security Agenda To Achieve a World Safe and Secure From Infectious Disease Threats), and is hereby reconvened as described in that order.

(c) Responsibility for National Biodefense Preparedness. Notwithstanding any statements in the National Security Presidential Memorandum-14 of September 18, 2018 (Support for National Biodefense), the APNSA shall be responsible for coordinating the Nation's biodefense preparedness efforts, and, as stated in sections 1 and 2 of this order, the COVID-19 Response Coordinator shall be responsible for coordinating the Federal Government's response to the COVID-19 pandemic.

Sec. 4. Prompt Resolution of Issues Related to the United States COVID-19 Response. The heads of agencies shall, as soon as practicable, bring any procedural, departmental, legal, or funding obstacle to the COVID-19

response to the attention of the COVID-19 Response Coordinator. The

COVID-19 Response Coordinator shall, in coordination with relevant agencies,

the APDP, and the APNSA, as appropriate, immediately bring to the President's

attention any issues that require Presidential guidance or decision-making.

Sec. 5. General Provisions. (a) Nothing in this order

shall be construed to impair or otherwise affect:

(i) the authority granted by law to an executive

department or agency, or the head thereof; or

(ii) the functions of the Director of the Office of Management and Budget

relating to budgetary, administrative, or legislative proposals.

(b) This order shall be implemented consistent with

applicable law and subject to availability of appropriations.

(c) This order is not intended to, and does not, create any right

or benefit, substantive or procedural, enforceable at law or in equity

by any party against the United States, its departments, agencies, or

entities, its officers, employees, or agents, or any other person.

THE WHITE HOUSE,

EXECUTIVE ORDER

PROTECTING THE FEDERAL WORKFORCE AND

REQUIRING MASK-WEARING

By the authority vested in me as President by the Constitution

and the laws of the United States of America, including section 7902(c)

of title 5, United States Code, it is hereby ordered as follows:

Section 1. Policy. It is the policy of my Administration to halt the spread

of coronavirus disease 2019 (COVID-19) by relying on the best available data and

science-based public health measures. Such measures include wearing masks when

around others, physical distancing, and other related precautions recommended

by the Centers for Disease Control and Prevention (CDC). Put simply, masks

and other public health measures reduce the spread of the disease, particularly

when communities make widespread use of such measures, and thus save lives.

Accordingly, to protect the Federal workforce and individuals

interacting with the Federal workforce, and to ensure the continuity of

Government services and activities, on-duty or on-site Federal employees,

on-site Federal contractors, and other individuals in Federal buildings and on Federal lands should all wear masks, maintain physical distance, and adhere to other public health measures, as provided in CDC guidelines.

Sec. 2. Immediate Action Regarding Federal Employees, Contractors, Buildings, and Lands. (a) The heads of executive departments and agencies (agencies) shall immediately take action, as appropriate and consistent with applicable law, to require compliance with CDC guidelines with respect to wearing masks, maintaining physical distance, and other public health measures by: on-duty or on-site Federal employees; on-site Federal contractors; and all persons in Federal buildings or on Federal lands.

(b) The Director of the Office of Management and Budget (OMB), the Director of the Office of Personnel Management (OPM), and the Administrator of General Services, in coordination with the President's Management Council and the Coordinator of the COVID-19 Response and Counselor to the President (COVID-19 Response Coordinator), shall promptly issue guidance to assist heads of agencies with implementation of this section.

(c) Heads of agencies shall promptly consult, as appropriate, with State, local, Tribal, and territorial government officials, Federal employees, Federal employee unions, Federal contractors, and any other interested parties concerning the implementation of this section.

(d) Heads of agencies may make categorical or case-by-case exceptions in implementing subsection (a) of this section to the extent that doing

so is necessary or required by law, and consistent with applicable law. If

heads of agencies make such exceptions, they shall require appropriate

alternative safeguards, such as additional physical distancing measures,

additional testing, or reconfiguration of workspace, consistent with applicable

law. Heads of agencies shall document all exceptions in writing.

(e) Heads of agencies shall review their existing authorities and, to the

extent permitted by law and subject to the availability of appropriations and

resources, seek to provide masks to individuals in Federal buildings when needed.

(f) The COVID-19 Response Coordinator shall coordinate the

implementation of this section. Heads of the agencies listed in 31 U.S.C. 901(b) shall

update the COVID-19 Response Coordinator on their progress in implementing this

section, including any categorical exceptions established under subsection (d) of

this section, within 7 days of the date of this order and regularly thereafter. Heads

of agencies are encouraged to bring to the attention of the COVID-19 Response

Coordinator any questions regarding the scope or implementation of this section.

Sec. 3. Encouraging Masking Across America. (a) The Secretary

of Health and Human Services (HHS), including through the Director of

CDC, shall engage, as appropriate, with State, local, Tribal, and territorial

officials, as well as business, union, academic, and other community leaders, regarding mask-wearing and other public health measures, with the goal

of maximizing public compliance with, and addressing any obstacles to,

mask-wearing and other public health best practices identified by CDC.

(b) The COVID-19 Response Coordinator, in coordination with

the Secretary of HHS, the Secretary of Homeland Security, and the

heads of other relevant agencies, shall promptly identify and inform

agencies of options to incentivize, support, and encourage widespread

mask-wearing consistent with CDC guidelines and applicable law.

Sec. 4. Safer Federal Workforce Task Force.

(a) Establishment. There is hereby established the

Safer Federal Workforce Task Force (Task Force).

(b) Membership. The Task Force shall consist of the following members:

(i) the Director of OPM, who shall serve as Co-Chair;

(ii) the Administrator of General Services, who shall serve as Co-Chair;

(iii) the COVID-19 Response Coordinator, who shall serve as Co-Chair;

(iv) the Director of OMB;

(v) the Director of the Federal Protective Service;

(vi) the Director of the United States Secret Service;

(vii) the Administrator of the Federal Emergency Management Agency;

(viii) the Director of CDC; and

(ix)   the heads of such other agencies as the Co-Chairs

may individually or jointly invite to participate.

(c) Organization. A member of the Task Force may designate, to perform

the Task Force functions of the member, a senior-level official who is a

full-time officer or employee of the member's agency. At the direction

of the Co-Chairs, the Task Force may establish subgroups consisting

exclusively of Task Force members or their designees, as appropriate.

(d) Administration. The General Services Administration shall provide funding

and administrative support for the Task Force to the extent permitted by law

and within existing appropriations. The Co-Chairs shall convene regular

meetings of the Task Force, determine its agenda, and direct its work.

(e) Mission. The Task Force shall provide ongoing guidance to heads

of agencies on the operation of the Federal Government, the safety of its

employees, and the continuity of Government functions during the COVID-19

pandemic. Such guidance shall be based on public health best practices as

determined by CDC and other public health experts, and shall address, at a

minimum, the following subjects as they relate to the Federal workforce:

(i)   testing methodologies and protocols;

(ii)   case investigation and contact tracing;

(iii) requirements of and limitations on physical distancing, including recommended occupancy and density standards;

(iv)   equipment needs and requirements, including personal protective equipment;

(v)   air filtration;

(vi)   enhanced environmental disinfection and cleaning;

(vii)   safe commuting and telework options;

(viii)   enhanced technological infrastructure to support telework;

(ix)   vaccine prioritization, distribution, and administration;

(x)   approaches for coordinating with State, local, Tribal, and territorial health

officials, as well as business, union, academic, and other community leaders;

(xi)   any management infrastructure needed by agencies

to implement public health guidance; and

(xii)   circumstances under which exemptions might

appropriately be made to agency policies in accordance with

CDC guidelines, such as for mission-critical purposes.

(f) Agency Cooperation. The head of each agency listed in 31 U.S.C. 901(b)

shall, consistent with applicable law, promptly provide the Task Force a report

on COVID-19 safety protocols, safety plans, or guidance regarding the operation

of the agency and the safety of its employees, and any other information

that the head of the agency deems relevant to the Task Force's work.

Sec. 5. Federal Employee Testing. The Secretary of HHS, through the Director of CDC, shall promptly develop and submit to the COVID-19 Response Coordinator a testing plan for the Federal workforce. This plan shall be based on community transmission metrics and address the populations to be tested, testing types, frequency of testing, positive case protocols, and coordination with local public health authorities for contact tracing.

Sec. 6. Research and Development. The Director of the Office of Science and Technology Policy, in consultation with the Secretary of HHS (through the National Science and Technology Council), the Director of OMB, the Director of CDC, the Director of the National Institutes of Health, the Director of the National Science Foundation, and the heads of any other appropriate agencies, shall assess the availability of Federal research grants to study best practices for implementing, and innovations to better implement, effective mask-wearing and physical distancing policies, with respect to both the Federal workforce and the general public.

Sec. 7. Scope. (a) For purposes of this order:

(i) "Federal employees" and "Federal contractors" mean employees (including members of the Armed Forces and members of the National Guard in Federal service) and contractors (including such contractors' employees) working for the executive branch;

(ii) "Federal buildings" means buildings, or office space within buildings, owned, rented, or leased by the executive branch of which a substantial portion of occupants are Federal employees or Federal contractors; and

(iii) "Federal lands" means lands under executive branch control.

(b) The Director of OPM and the Administrator of General Services shall seek to consult, in coordination with the heads of any other relevant agencies and the COVID-19 Response Coordinator, with the Sergeants at Arms of the Senate and the House of Representatives and the Director of the Administrative Office of the United States Courts (or such other persons designated by the Majority and Minority Leaders of the Senate, the Speaker and Minority Leader of the House, or the Chief Justice of the United States, respectively), to promote mask-wearing, physical distancing, and adherence to other public health measures within the legislative and judicial branches, and shall provide requested technical assistance as needed to facilitate compliance with CDC guidelines.

Sec. 8. General Provisions. (a) Nothing in this order shall be construed to impair or otherwise affect:

(i) the authority granted by law to an executive department or agency, or the head thereof; or

(ii) the functions of the Director of the Office of Management and Budget relating to budgetary, administrative, or legislative proposals.

(b) This order shall be implemented consistent with applicable law and subject to the availability of appropriations.

(c) Independent agencies are strongly encouraged to

comply with the requirements of this order.

(d) This order is not intended to, and does not, create any right or

benefit, substantive or procedural, enforceable at law or in equity

by any party against the United States, its departments, agencies, or

entities, its officers, employees, or agents, or any other person.

THE WHITE HOUSE,

EXECUTIVE ORDER

ESTABLISHING THE COVID-19 PANDEMIC TESTING BOARD AND ENSURING A SUSTAINABLE PUBLIC HEALTH WORKFORCE FOR COVID-19 AND OTHER BIOLOGICAL THREATS

By the authority vested in me as President by the Constitution and the laws of the United States of America, including section 301 of title 3, United States Code, it is hereby ordered as follows:

Section 1. Policy. It is the policy of my Administration to control coronavirus disease 2019 (COVID-19) by using a Government-wide, unified approach that includes: establishing a national COVID-19 testing and public health workforce strategy; working to expand the supply of tests; working to bring test manufacturing to the United States, where possible; working to enhance laboratory testing capacity; working to expand the public health workforce; supporting screening testing for schools and priority populations; and ensuring a clarity of messaging about the use of tests and insurance coverage.

Sec. 2. COVID-19 Pandemic Testing Board.

(a) Establishment and Membership. There is established a COVID-19

Pandemic Testing Board (Testing Board), chaired by the Coordinator of the COVID-19 Response and Counselor to the President (COVID-19 Response Coordinator) or his designee. The Testing Board shall include representatives from executive departments and agencies (agencies) that are designated by the President. The heads of agencies so designated shall designate officials from their respective agencies to represent them on the Testing Board.

(b) Mission and Functions. To support the implementation and oversight of the policy laid out in section 1 of this order, the Testing Board shall:

(i) coordinate Federal Government efforts to promote COVID-19 diagnostic, screening, and surveillance testing;

(ii) make recommendations to the President with respect to prioritizing the Federal Government's assistance to State, local, Tribal, and territorial authorities, in order to expand testing and reduce disparities in access to testing;

(iii) identify barriers to access and use of testing in, and coordinate Federal Government efforts to increase testing for:

(A) priority populations, including healthcare workers and other essential workers;

(B) communities with major shortages in testing availability and use;

(C) at-risk settings, including long-term care facilities, correctional facilities, immigration custodial settings, detention facilities, schools, child care settings, and food processing and manufacturing facilities; and

(D) high-risk groups, including people experiencing

homelessness, migrants, and seasonal workers;

(iv) identify methods to expand State, local, Tribal, and territorial

capacity to conduct testing, contact tracing, and isolation and quarantine,

in order for schools, businesses, and travel to be conducted safely;

(v) provide guidance on how to enhance the clarity, consistency,

and transparency of Federal Government communication with

the public about the goals and purposes of testing;

(vi) identify options for the Federal Government to maximize

testing capacity of commercial labs and academic labs; and

(vii) propose short- and long-term reforms for the Federal Government to:

increase State, local, Tribal, and territorial capacity to conduct testing; expand

genomic sequencing; and improve the effectiveness and speed of the Federal

Government's response to future pandemics and other biological emergencies.

(d) The Chair of the Testing Board shall coordinate with the Secretary of Health

and Human Services (HHS) and the heads of other relevant agencies or their

designees, as necessary, to ensure that the Testing Board's work is coordinated

with the Public Health Emergency Countermeasures Enterprise within HHS.

Sec. 3. Actions to Address the Cost of COVID-19 Testing. (a) The

Secretary of the Treasury, the Secretary of HHS, and the Secretary of

Labor, in coordination with the COVID-19 Response Coordinator, shall

promptly, and as appropriate and consistent with applicable law:

(i) facilitate the provision of COVID-19 testing free of charge

to those who lack comprehensive health insurance; and

(ii) clarify group health plans' and health insurance issuers'

obligations to provide coverage for COVID-19 testing.

(b) The Secretary of HHS, the Secretary of Education, and the Secretary of

Homeland Security, through the Administrator of the Federal Emergency

Management Agency (FEMA), in coordination with the COVID-19 Response

Coordinator, shall promptly, and as appropriate and consistent with applicable law:

(i) provide support for surveillance tests for settings such as schools; and

(ii) expand equitable access to COVID-19 testing.

Sec. 4. Establishing a Public Health Workforce Program. (a) The

Secretary of HHS and the Secretary of Labor shall promptly consult with

State, local, Tribal, and territorial leaders to understand the challenges

they face in pandemic response efforts, including challenges recruiting

and training sufficient personnel to ensure adequate and equitable

community-based testing, and testing in schools and high-risk settings.

(b) The Secretary of HHS shall, as appropriate and

consistent with applicable law, as soon as practicable:

(i)   provide technical support to State, local, Tribal, and territorial public health agencies with respect to testing and contact-tracing efforts; and

(ii) assist such authorities in the training of public health workers. This may include technical assistance to non-Federal public health workforces in connection with testing, contact tracing, and mass vaccinations, as well as other urgent public health workforce needs, such as combating opioid use.

(c) The Secretary of HHS shall submit to the President, through the COVID-19 Response Coordinator, the Assistant to the President for Domestic Policy (APDP), and the Assistant to the President for National Security Affairs (APNSA), a plan detailing:

(i)   how the Secretary of HHS would deploy personnel in response to future high-consequence public health threats; and

(ii) five-year targets and budget requirements for achieving a sustainable public health workforce, as well as options for expanding HHS capacity, such as by expanding the U.S. Public Health Service Commissioned Corps and Epidemic Intelligence Service, so that the Department can better respond to future pandemics and other biological threats.

(d) The Secretary of HHS, the Secretary of Homeland Security, the Secretary of Labor, the Secretary of Education, and the Chief Executive Officer of the Corporation for National and Community Service, in coordination with the

COVID-19 Response Coordinator, the APDP, and the APNSA, shall submit a plan to the President for establishing a national contact tracing and COVID-19 public health workforce program, to be known as the U.S. Public Health Job Corps, which shall be modeled on or developed as a component of the FEMA Corps program. Such plan shall include means by which the U.S. Public Health Job Corps can be part of the National Civilian Community Corps program, as well as recommendations about whether it would be appropriate for the U.S. Public Health Job Corps to immediately assign personnel from any of the agencies involved in the creation of the plan, including existing AmeriCorps members, to join or aid the U.S. Public Health Job Corps. The U.S. Public Health Job Corps will:

(i) conduct and train individuals in contact tracing related to the COVID-19 pandemic;

(ii) assist in outreach for vaccination efforts, including by administering vaccination clinics;

(iii) assist with training programs for State, local, Tribal, and territorial governments to provide testing, including in schools; and

(iv) provide other necessary services to Americans affected by the COVID-19 pandemic.

Sec. 5. General Provisions. (a) Nothing in this order shall be construed to impair or otherwise affect:

(i) the authority granted by law to an executive

department or agency, or the head thereof; or

(ii) the functions of the Director of the Office of Management and Budget

relating to budgetary, administrative, or legislative proposals.

(b) This order shall be implemented consistent with applicable

law and subject to the availability of appropriations.

(c) This order is not intended to, and does not, create any right or

benefit, substantive or procedural, enforceable at law or in equity

by any party against the United States, its departments, agencies, or

entities, its officers, employees, or agents, or any other person.

THE WHITE HOUSE,
EXECUTIVE ORDER

IMPROVING AND EXPANDING ACCESS TO CARE AND TREATMENTS FOR COVID-19

By the authority vested in me as President by the Constitution and the laws of the United States of America, it is hereby ordered as follows:

Section 1. Policy. It is the policy of my Administration to improve the capacity of the Nation's healthcare systems to address coronavirus disease 2019 (COVID-19), to accelerate the development of novel therapies to treat COVID-19, and to improve all Americans' access to quality and affordable healthcare.

Sec. 2. Accelerating the Development of Novel Therapies. To enhance the Nation's ability to quickly develop the most promising COVID-19 interventions, the Secretary of Health and Human Services (HHS), in consultation with the Director of the National Institutes of Health, shall:

(a) develop a plan for supporting a range of studies, including large-scale randomized trials, for identifying optimal clinical management strategies, and for supporting the most promising treatments for COVID-19 and future high-consequence public health threats, that can be easily manufactured, distributed, and administered, both domestically and internationally;

(b) develop a plan, in consultation with non-governmental

partners, as appropriate, to support research:

(i) in rural hospitals and other rural locations; and

(ii) that studies the emerging evidence concerning the long-

term impact of COVID-19 on patient health; and

(c) consider steps to ensure that clinical trials include populations

that have been historically underrepresented in such trials.

Sec. 3. Improving the Capacity of the Nation's Healthcare Systems

to Address COVID-19. To bolster the capacity of the Nation's

healthcare systems to support healthcare workers and patients:

(a) The Secretary of Defense, the Secretary of HHS, the Secretary of Veterans

Affairs, and the heads of other relevant executive departments and agencies

(agencies), in coordination with the Coordinator of the COVID-19 Response

and Counselor to the President (COVID-19 Response Coordinator), shall

promptly, as appropriate and consistent with applicable law, provide targeted

surge assistance to critical care and long-term care facilities, including

nursing homes and skilled nursing facilities, assisted living facilities,

intermediate care facilities for individuals with disabilities, and residential

treatment centers, in their efforts to combat the spread of COVID-19.

(b) The COVID-19 Response Coordinator, in coordination with the Secretary of Defense, the Secretary of HHS, the Secretary of Veterans Affairs, and the heads of other relevant agencies, shall review the needs of Federal facilities providing care to COVID-19 patients and develop recommendations for further actions such facilities can take to support active military personnel, veterans, and Tribal nations during this crisis.

(c) The Secretary of HHS shall promptly:

(i) issue recommendations on how States and healthcare providers can increase the capacity of their healthcare workforces to address the COVID-19 pandemic; and

(ii) through the Administrator of the Health Resources and Services Administration and the Administrator of the Substance Abuse and Mental Health Services Administration, take appropriate actions, as consistent with applicable law, to expand access to programs and services designed to meet the long-term health needs of patients recovering from COVID-19, including through technical assistance and support to community health centers.

Sec. 4. Improving Access to Quality and Affordable Healthcare. (a) To facilitate the equitable and effective distribution of therapeutics and bolster clinical care capacity where needed to support patient care, the Secretary of Defense, the Secretary of HHS, and the Secretary of Veterans Affairs, in coordination with the COVID-19 Response Coordinator, shall establish targets for the production, allocation, and distribution of COVID-19 treatments. To meet those targets, the Secretary of Defense, the Secretary of HHS, and the Secretary of Veterans Affairs shall consider prioritizing, including through grants for research and development, investments in therapeutics that can be readily administered and scaled.

(b) To facilitate the utilization of existing COVID-19 treatments, the Secretary of HHS shall identify barriers to maximizing the effective and equitable use of existing COVID-19 treatments and shall, as appropriate and consistent with applicable law, provide support to State, local, Tribal, and territorial authorities aimed at overcoming those barriers.

(c) To address the affordability of treatments and clinical care, the Secretary of HHS shall, promptly and as appropriate and consistent with applicable law:

(i) evaluate the COVID-19 Uninsured Program, operated by the Health Resources and Services Administration within HHS, and take any available steps to promote access to treatments and clinical care for those without adequate coverage, to support safety-net providers in delivering such treatments and clinical care, and to make the Program easy to use and accessible for patients and providers, with information about the Program widely disseminated; and

(ii) evaluate Medicare, Medicaid, group health plans, and health insurance issuers, and take any available steps to promote insurance coverage for safe and effective COVID-19 treatments and clinical care.

Sec. 5. General Provisions. (a) Nothing in this order shall be construed to impair or otherwise affect:

(i) the authority granted by law to an executive department or agency, or the head thereof; or

(ii) the functions of the Director of the Office of Management and Budget relating to budgetary, administrative, or legislative proposals.

(b) This order shall be implemented consistent with applicable law and subject to the availability of appropriations.

(c) This order is not intended to, and does not, create any right or benefit, substantive or procedural, enforceable at law or in equity by any party against the United States, its departments, agencies, or entities, its officers, employees, or agents, or any other person.

THE WHITE HOUSE,

EXECUTIVE ORDER

ENSURING A DATA-DRIVEN RESPONSE

TO COVID-19 AND FUTURE HIGH-CONSEQUENCE

PUBLIC HEALTH THREATS

By the authority vested in me as President by the Constitution and the laws of the United States of America, it is hereby ordered as follows:

Section 1. Policy. It is the policy of this Administration to respond to the coronavirus disease 2019 (COVID-19) pandemic through effective approaches guided by the best available science and data, including by building back a better public health infrastructure. This stronger public health infrastructure must help the Nation effectively prevent, detect, and respond to future biological threats, both domestically and internationally.

Consistent with this policy, the heads of all executive departments and agencies (agencies) shall facilitate the gathering, sharing, and publication of COVID-19-related data, in coordination with the Coordinator of the COVID-19 Response and Counselor to the President (COVID-19 Response Coordinator), to the extent permitted by law, and with appropriate protections for confidentiality, privacy, law enforcement, and national security. These efforts shall assist Federal, State, local, Tribal, and territorial authorities in developing and implementing policies to facilitate informed community decision-making, to further public understanding of the pandemic and the response, and to deter the spread of misinformation and disinformation.

Sec. 2. Enhancing Data Collection and Collaboration Capabilities for High-Consequence Public Health Threats, Such as the COVID-19 Pandemic. (a) The Secretary of Defense, the Attorney General, the Secretary of Commerce, the Secretary of Labor, the Secretary of Health and Human Services (HHS), the Secretary of Education, the Director of the Office of Management and Budget (OMB), the Director of National Intelligence, the Director of the Office of Science and Technology Policy (OSTP), and the Director of the National Science Foundation shall each promptly designate a senior official to serve as their agency's lead to work on COVID-19- and pandemic-related data issues. This official, in consultation with the COVID-19 Response Coordinator, shall take steps to make data relevant to high-consequence public health threats, such as the COVID-19 pandemic, publicly available and accessible.

(b) The COVID-19 Response Coordinator shall, as necessary, convene appropriate representatives from relevant agencies to coordinate the agencies' collection, provision, and analysis of data, including key equity indicators, regarding the COVID-19 response, as well as their sharing

of such data with State, local, Tribal, and territorial authorities.

(c) The Director of OMB, in consultation with the Director of OSTP, the

United States Chief Technology Officer, and the COVID-19 Response Coordinator,

shall promptly review the Federal Government's existing approaches to open

data, and shall issue supplemental guidance, as appropriate and consistent with

applicable law, concerning how to de-identify COVID-19-related data; how

to make data open to the public in human- and machine-readable formats as

rapidly as possible; and any other topic the Director of OMB concludes would

appropriately advance the policy of this order. Any guidance shall include

appropriate protections for the information described in section 5 of this order.

(d) The Director of the Office of Personnel Management,

in consultation with the Director of OMB, shall promptly:

(i) review the ability of agencies to hire personnel expeditiously

into roles related to information technology and the collection,

provision, analysis, or other use of data to address high-consequence

public health threats, such as the COVID-19 pandemic; and

(ii) take action, as appropriate and consistent with

applicable law, to support agencies in such efforts.

Sec. 3. Public Health Data Systems. The Secretary of

HHS, in consultation with the COVID-19 Response Coordinator and the heads of relevant agencies, shall promptly:

(a) review the effectiveness, interoperability, and connectivity of public health data systems supporting the detection of and response to high-consequence public health threats, such as the COVID-19 pandemic;

(b) review the collection of morbidity and mortality data by State, local, Tribal, and territorial governments during high-consequence public health threats, such as the COVID-19 pandemic; and

(c) issue a report summarizing the findings of the reviews detailed in subsections (a) and (b) of this section and any recommendations for addressing areas for improvement identified in the reviews.

Sec. 4. Advancing Innovation in Public Health Data and Analytics. The Director of OSTP, in coordination with the National Science and Technology Council, as appropriate, shall develop a plan for advancing innovation in public health data and analytics in the United States.

Sec. 5. Privileged Information. Nothing in this order shall compel or authorize the disclosure of privileged information, law-enforcement information, national-security information, personal information, or information the disclosure of which is prohibited by law.

Sec. 6. General Provisions. (a) Nothing in this order

shall be construed to impair or otherwise affect:

(i) the authority granted by law to an executive

department or agency, or the head thereof; or

(ii) the functions of the Director of the Office of Management and Budget

relating to budgetary, administrative, or legislative proposals.

(b) This order shall be implemented consistent with

applicable law and subject to the availability of appropriations.

(c) This order is not intended to, and does not, create any right or

benefit, substantive or procedural, enforceable at law or in equity

by any party against the United States, its departments, agencies, or

entities, its officers, employees, or agents, or any other person.

THE WHITE HOUSE,

EXECUTIVE ORDER

A SUSTAINABLE PUBLIC HEALTH SUPPLY CHAIN

By the authority vested in me as President by the Constitution and the

laws of the United States of America, including the Defense Production Act

of 1950, as amended (50 U.S.C. 4501 et seq.), sections 319 and 361 of the Public

Health Service Act (42 U.S.C. 247d and 264), sections 306 and 307 of the Robert T.

Stafford Disaster Relief and Emergency Assistance Act (42 U.S.C. 5149 and 5150),

and section 301 of title 3, United States Code, it is hereby ordered as follows:

Section 1. Purpose. The Federal Government must act urgently and

effectively to combat the coronavirus disease 2019 (COVID-19) pandemic. To

that end, this order directs immediate actions to secure supplies necessary

for responding to the pandemic, so that those supplies are available, and

remain available, to the Federal Government and State, local, Tribal, and

territorial authorities, as well as to America's health care workers, health

systems, and patients. These supplies are vital to the Nation's ability

to reopen its schools and economy as soon and safely as possible.

Sec. 2. Immediate Inventory of Response Supplies and Identification of Emergency Needs. (a) The Secretary of State, the Secretary of Defense, the Secretary of Health and Human Services, the Secretary of Homeland Security, and the heads of appropriate executive departments and agencies (agencies), in coordination with the COVID-19 Response Coordinator, shall:

(i) immediately review the availability of critical materials, treatments, and supplies needed to combat COVID-19 (pandemic response supplies), including personal protective equipment (PPE) and the resources necessary to effectively produce and distribute tests and vaccines at scale; and

(ii) assess, including by reviewing prior such assessments, whether United States industry can be reasonably expected to provide such supplies in a timely manner.

(b) Where a review and assessment described in section 2(a)

(i) of this order identifies shortfalls in the provision of pandemic response supplies, the head of the relevant agency shall:

(i) promptly revise its operational assumptions and planning factors being used to determine the scope and prioritization, acquisition, and distribution of such supplies; and

(ii) take appropriate action using all available legal authorities, including the Defense Production Act, to fill those shortfalls as soon as practicable by acquiring additional stockpiles, improving distribution systems, building market capacity, or expanding the industrial base.

(c) Upon completing the review and assessment described in section 2(a)(i) of this order, the Secretary of Health and Human Services shall provide to the President, through the COVID-19 Response Coordinator, a report on the status and inventory of the Strategic National Stockpile.

(d) The Secretary of State, the Secretary of Defense, the Secretary of Health and Human Services, the Secretary of Homeland Security, and the heads of any other agencies relevant to inventorying pandemic response supplies shall, as soon as practicable, provide to the President, through the COVID-19 Response Coordinator, a report consisting of:

(i)   an assessment of the need for, and an inventory of current supplies of, key pandemic response supplies;

(ii) an analysis of their agency's capacity to produce, provide, and distribute pandemic response supplies;

(iii) an assessment of their agency's procurement of pandemic response supplies on the availability of such supplies on the open market;

(iv) an account of all existing or ongoing agency actions, contracts, and investment agreements regarding pandemic response supplies;

(v)   a list of any gaps between the needs identified in section 2(a)(i) of this order and supply chain delivery, and recommendations on how to close such gaps; and

(vi) a compilation and summary of their agency's existing distribution and prioritization plans for pandemic response supplies, which shall include

any assumptions or planning factors used to determine such needs and

any recommendations for changes to such assumptions or factors.

(e) The COVID-19 Response Coordinator, in coordination with the

heads of appropriate agencies, shall review the report described in section 2(d)

of this order and submit recommendations to the President that address:

(i) whether additional use of the Defense Production Act, by the President or

agencies exercising delegated authority under the Act, would be helpful; and

(ii) the extent to which liability risk, regulatory requirements, or

other factors impede the development, production, and procurement

of pandemic response supplies, and any actions that can be taken,

consistent with law, to remove those impediments.

(f) The heads of agencies responsible for completing the

requirements of this section, as appropriate and in coordination with

the COVID-19 Response Coordinator, shall consult with State, local,

Tribal, and territorial authorities, as well as with other entities critical to

assessing the availability of and need for pandemic response supplies.

Sec. 3. Pricing. To take steps to address the

pricing of pandemic response supplies:

(a) The Secretary of Health and Human Services shall promptly recommend to the President, through the COVID-19 Response Coordinator,

whether any changes should be made to the authorities delegated to the

Secretary by Executive Order 13910 of March 23, 2020 (Preventing Hoarding

of Health and Medical Resources To Respond to the Spread of COVID-19),

with respect to scarce materials or materials the supply of which would be

threatened by accumulation for the purpose of hoarding or price gouging.

(b) The Secretary of Defense, the Secretary of Health and Human

Services, and the Secretary of Homeland Security shall promptly review

and provide to the President, through the COVID-19 Response Coordinator,

recommendations for how to address the pricing of pandemic response

supplies, including whether and how to direct the use of reasonable pricing

clauses in Federal contracts and investment agreements, or other related

vehicles, and whether to use General Services Administration Schedules to

facilitate State, local, Tribal, and territorial government buyers and compacts

in purchasing pandemic response supplies using Federal supply schedules.

Sec. 4. Pandemic Supply Chain Resilience Strategy. Within 180 days

of the date of this order, the Secretary of Defense, the Secretary of Health and

Human Services, and the Secretary of Homeland Security, in coordination with

the Assistant to the President for National Security Affairs (APNSA), the Assistant

to the President for Domestic Policy, the COVID-19 Response Coordinator, and the heads of any agencies or entities selected by the APNSA and COVID-19 Response Coordinator, shall provide to the President a strategy to design, build, and sustain a long-term capability in the United States to manufacture supplies for future pandemics and biological threats. This strategy shall include:

(a) mechanisms to respond to emergency supply needs of State, local, Tribal, and territorial authorities, which should include standards and processes to prioritize requests and delivery and to ensure equitable distribution based on public health criteria;

(b) an analysis of the role of foreign supply chains in America's pandemic supply chain, America's role in the international public health supply chain, and options for strengthening and better coordinating global supply chain systems in future pandemics;

(c) mechanisms to address points of failure in the supply chains and to ensure necessary redundancies;

(d) the roles of the Strategic National Stockpile and other Federal and military stockpiles in providing pandemic supplies on an ongoing or emergency basis, including their roles in allocating supplies across States, localities, tribes, and territories, sustaining supplies during a pandemic, and in contingency planning to ensure adequate preparedness for future pandemics and public health emergencies;

(e) approaches to assess and maximize the value and

efficacy of public/private partnerships and the value of Federal

investments in latent manufacturing capacity; and

(f) an approach to develop a multi-year implementation

plan for domestic production of pandemic supplies.

Sec. 5. Access to Strategic National Stockpile. The Secretary of Health and

Human Services shall consult with Tribal authorities and take steps, as appropriate

and consistent with applicable law, to facilitate access to the Strategic National

Stockpile for federally recognized Tribal governments, Indian Health Service

healthcare providers, Tribal health authorities, and Urban Indian Organizations.

Sec. 6. General Provisions. (a) Nothing in this order

shall be construed to impair or otherwise affect:

(i) the authority granted by law to an executive

department or agency, or the head thereof; or

(ii) the functions of the Director of the Office of Management and Budget

relating to budgetary, administrative, or legislative proposals.

(b) This order shall be implemented consistent with

applicable law and subject to the availability of appropriations.

(c) This order is not intended to, and does not, create any right

or benefit, substantive or procedural, enforceable at law or in equity

by any party against the United States, its departments, agencies, or

entities, its officers, employees, or agents, or any other person.

THE WHITE HOUSE,

MEMORANDUM FOR THE SECRETARY OF DEFENSE

THE SECRETARY OF HOMELAND

SECURITY

SUBJECT: Memorandum to Extend Federal Support to

Governors' Use of the National Guard to Respond

to COVID-19 and to Increase Reimbursement and

Other Assistance Provided to States

By the authority vested in me as President by the Constitution and the laws

of the United States of America, including the Robert T. Stafford Disaster

Relief and Emergency Assistance Act, 42 U.S.C. 5121–5207 (the "Stafford Act"),

and section 502 of title 32, United States Code, I hereby order as follows:

Section 1. Policy. Consistent with the nationwide emergency declaration

concerning the coronavirus disease 2019 (COVID-19) pandemic on March 13,

2020, it is the policy of my Administration to combat and respond to COVID-19

with the full capacity and capability of the Federal Government to protect and support our families, schools, and businesses, and to assist State, local, Tribal, and territorial governments to do the same, to the extent authorized by law.

Sec. 2. Support of Operations or Missions to Prevent and Respond to the Spread of COVID-19. (a) The Secretary of Defense shall, to the maximum extent feasible and consistent with mission requirements (including geographic proximity), request pursuant to 32 U.S.C. 502(f) that all State and territorial governors order National Guard forces to perform duty to fulfill mission assignments, on a fully reimbursable basis, that the Federal Emergency Management Agency (FEMA) issues to the Department of Defense for the purpose of supporting State, local, Tribal, and territorial emergency assistance efforts under the Stafford Act.

(b) FEMA shall fund 100 percent of the cost of activities associated with all mission assignments for the use of the National Guard under 32 U.S.C. 502(f) to respond to COVID-19, as authorized by sections 403 (42 U.S.C. 5170b), 502 (42 U.S.C. 5192), and 503 (42 U.S.C. 5193) of the Stafford Act.

(c) This section supersedes prior Presidential Memoranda requesting the use of the National Guard to respond to the COVID-19 emergency to the extent they are inconsistent with this memorandum.

Sec. 3. Assistance for Category B Emergency Protective Measures. (a) In accordance with sections 403 (42 U.S.C. 5170b) and 502 (42 U.S.C. 5192) of the Stafford Act, FEMA shall, as appropriate and consistent with applicable law, make available under Category B of the Public Assistance program such assistance as may be required by States (including territories and the District of Columbia), local governments, and Tribal governments to provide for the safe opening and operation of eligible schools, child-care facilities, healthcare facilities, non-congregate shelters, domestic violence shelters, transit systems, and other eligible applicants. Such assistance may include funding for the provision of personal protective equipment and disinfecting services and supplies.

(b) FEMA shall make assistance under this section available at a 100 percent Federal cost share until September 30, 2021.

Sec. 4. Advanced Reimbursement. To make reimbursements for approved work under the Stafford Act to respond to COVID-19 available more quickly, FEMA shall expedite reimbursement for eligible emergency work projects and, as appropriate and consistent with applicable law, provide an advance of the Federal share on a percentage of the expected reimbursement from FEMA-approved projects.

Sec. 5. One-Hundred Percent Cost Share Termination. The 100 percent Federal cost share for use of National Guard forces authorized by section 2(b) of this memorandum shall extend to, and shall be available for, orders of any length authorizing duty through September 30, 2021.

Sec. 6. General Provisions. (a) Nothing in this memorandum shall be construed to impair or otherwise affect:

(i) the authority granted by law to an executive department or agency, or the head thereof; or

(ii) the functions of the Director of the Office of Management and Budget relating to budgetary, administrative, or legislative proposals.

(b) This memorandum shall be implemented consistent with applicable law and subject to the availability of appropriations.

(c) This memorandum is not intended to, and does not, create

any right or benefit, substantive or procedural, enforceable at law or in

equity by any party against the United States, its departments, agencies,

or entities, its officers, employees, or agents, or any other person.

(d) The Secretary of Defense is authorized and directed

to publish this memorandum in the Federal Register.

EXECUTIVE ORDER

SUPPORTING THE REOPENING AND CONTINUING OPERATION OF SCHOOLS AND EARLY CHILDHOOD EDUCATION PROVIDERS

By the authority vested in me as President by the Constitution and the laws of the United States of America, to ensure that students receive a high-quality education during the coronavirus disease 2019 (COVID-19) pandemic, and to support the safe reopening and continued operation of schools, child care providers, Head Start programs, and institutions of higher education, it is hereby ordered as follows:

Section 1. Policy. Every student in America deserves a high-quality education in a safe environment. This promise, which was already out of reach for too many, has been further threatened by the COVID-19 pandemic. School and higher education administrators, educators, faculty, child care providers, custodians and other staff, and families have gone above and beyond to support children's and students' learning and meet their needs during this crisis. Students and teachers alike have found new ways to teach and learn. Many child care providers continue to provide care and learning opportunities to children in homes and centers across the country. However, leadership and support from the Federal Government is needed. Two principles should guide the Federal Government's response to the COVID-19 crisis with respect to schools, child care providers, Head Start programs, and higher education institutions. First, the health and safety of children, students, educators, families, and communities is paramount. Second, every student in the United States should have the opportunity to receive a high-quality education, during and beyond the pandemic.

Accordingly, it is the policy of my Administration to provide support to help create the conditions for safe, in-person learning as quickly as possible; ensure high-quality instruction and the delivery of essential services often received by students and young children at school, institutions of higher education, child care providers, and Head Start programs; mitigate learning loss caused by the pandemic; and address educational disparities and inequities that the pandemic has created and exacerbated.

Sec. 2. Agency Roles and Responsibilities. The following assignments of responsibility shall be exercised in furtherance of the policy described in section 1 of this order:

(a) The Secretary of Education shall, consistent with applicable law:

(i)   provide, in consultation with the Secretary of Health and Human Services, evidence-based guidance to assist States and elementary and secondary schools in deciding whether and how to reopen, and how to remain open, for in-person learning; and in safely conducting in-person learning, including by implementing mitigation measures such as cleaning, masking, proper ventilation, and testing;

(ii)　provide, in consultation with the Secretary of Health and Human Services, evidence-based guidance to institutions of higher education on safely reopening for in-person learning, which shall take into account considerations such as the institution's setting, resources, and the population it serves;

(iii)　provide advice to State, local, Tribal, and territorial educational authorities, institutions of higher education, local education agencies, and elementary and secondary schools regarding distance and online learning, blended learning, and in-person learning; and the promotion of mental health, social-emotional well-being, and communication with parents and families;

(iv)　develop a Safer Schools and Campuses Best Practices Clearinghouse to enable schools and institutions of higher education to share lessons learned and best practices for operating safely during the pandemic;

(v)　provide technical assistance to schools and institutions of higher education so that they can ensure high-quality learning during the pandemic;

(vi)　direct the Department of Education's Assistant Secretary for Civil Rights to deliver a report as soon as practicable on the disparate impacts of COVID-19 on students in elementary, secondary, and higher education, including those attending historically black colleges and universities, Tribal colleges and universities,

Hispanic-serving institutions, and other minority-serving institutions;

(vii)   coordinate with the Director of the Institute of Education Sciences

to facilitate, consistent with applicable law, the collection of data necessary

to fully understand the impact of the COVID-19 pandemic on students

and educators, including data on the status of in-person learning. These

data shall be disaggregated by student demographics, including race,

ethnicity, disability, English-language-learner status, and free or reduced

lunch status or other appropriate indicators of family income; and

(viii) consult with those who have been struggling for months with

the enormous challenges the COVID-19 pandemic poses for education,

including students; educators; unions; families; State, local, Tribal,

and territorial officials; and members of civil rights and disability

rights organizations, in carrying out the directives in this order.

   (b) The Secretary of Health and Human Services

shall, consistent with applicable law:

(i)   facilitate the collection of data needed to inform the safe reopening and

continued operation of elementary and secondary schools, child care providers, and

Head Start programs, and ensure that such data are readily available to State, local,

Tribal, and territorial leaders and the public, consistent with privacy interests, and

that such data are disaggregated by race, ethnicity, and other factors as appropriate;

(ii)   ensure, in coordination with the Coordinator of the COVID-19 Response and Counselor to the President (COVID-19 Response Coordinator) and other relevant agencies, that COVID-19-related supplies the Secretary administers, including testing materials, are equitably allocated to elementary and secondary schools, child care providers, and Head Start programs to support in-person care and learning;

(iii) to the maximum extent possible, support the development and operation of contact tracing programs at the State, local, Tribal, and territorial level, by providing guidance and technical support to ensure that contact tracing is available to facilitate the reopening and safe operation of elementary and secondary schools, child care providers, Head Start programs, and institutions of higher education;

(iv)   provide guidance needed for child care providers and Head Start programs for safely reopening and operating, including procedures for mitigation measures such as cleaning, masking, proper ventilation, and testing, as well as guidance related to meeting the needs of children, families, and staff who have been affected by the COVID-19 pandemic, including trauma-informed care, behavioral and mental health support, and family support, as appropriate; and

(v)   provide technical assistance to States, localities, Tribes, and territories to support the accelerated distribution of Federal COVID-19 relief funds to child care providers, and identify strategies to help child care providers safely remain open during the pandemic and beyond while the sector experiences widespread financial disruption due to increased costs and less revenue.

(c) The Secretary of Education and the Secretary of Health and Human Services shall submit a report to the Assistant to the President for Domestic Policy and the COVID-19 Response Coordinator identifying strategies to address the impact of COVID-19 on educational outcomes, especially along racial and socioeconomic lines, and shall share those strategies with State, local, Tribal, and territorial officials. In developing these strategies, the Secretaries shall, as appropriate and consistent with applicable law, consult with such officials, as well as with education experts; educators; unions; civil rights advocates; Tribal education experts; public health experts; child development experts; early educators, including child care providers; Head Start staff; school technology practitioners; foundations; families; students; community advocates; and others.

(d) The Federal Communications Commission is encouraged, consistent with applicable law, to increase connectivity options for students lacking reliable home broadband, so that they can continue to learn if their schools are operating remotely.

Sec. 3. General Provisions. (a) Nothing in this order shall be construed to impair or otherwise affect:

(i) the authority granted by law to an executive department or agency, or the head thereof; or

(ii) the functions of the Director of the Office of Management and Budget relating to budgetary, administrative, or legislative proposals.

(b) This order shall be implemented consistent with applicable law and subject to the availability of appropriations.

(c) This order is not intended to, and does not, create any right or benefit, substantive or procedural, enforceable at law or in equity by any party against the United States, its departments, agencies, or entities, its officers, employees, or agents, or any other person.

EXECUTIVE ORDER

PROTECTING WORKER HEALTH AND SAFETY

By the authority vested in me as President by the Constitution and the laws of the United States of America, it is hereby ordered as follows:

Section 1. Policy. Ensuring the health and safety of workers is a national priority and a moral imperative. Healthcare workers and other essential workers, many of whom are people of color and immigrants, have put their lives on the line during the coronavirus disease 2019 (COVID-19) pandemic. It is the policy of my Administration to protect the health and safety of workers from COVID-19.

The Federal Government must take swift action to reduce the risk that workers may contract COVID-19 in the workplace. That will require issuing science-based guidance to help keep workers safe from COVID-19 exposure, including with respect to mask-wearing; partnering with State and local governments to better protect public employees; enforcing worker health and safety requirements; and pushing for additional resources to help employers protect employees.

Sec. 2. Protecting Workers from COVID-19 Under the Occupational Safety and Health Act. The Secretary of Labor, acting through the Assistant Secretary of Labor for Occupational Safety and Health, in furtherance of the policy described in section 1 of this order and consistent with applicable law, shall:

(a) issue, within 2 weeks of the date of this order and in conjunction

or consultation with the heads of any other appropriate executive

departments and agencies (agencies), revised guidance to employers

on workplace safety during the COVID-19 pandemic;

(b) consider whether any emergency temporary standards on COVID-19,

including with respect to masks in the workplace, are necessary, and if such

standards are determined to be necessary, issue them by March 15, 2021;

(c) review the enforcement efforts of the Occupational Safety and

Health Administration (OSHA) related to COVID-19 and identify

any short-, medium-, and long-term changes that could be made to

better protect workers and ensure equity in enforcement;

(d) launch a national program to focus OSHA enforcement efforts

related to COVID-19 on violations that put the largest number of workers

at serious risk or are contrary to anti-retaliation principles; and

(e) coordinate with the Department of Labor's Office of Public Affairs and Office

of Public Engagement and all regional OSHA offices to conduct, consistent with

applicable law, a   multilingual outreach campaign to inform workers and

their representatives of their rights under applicable law. This campaign shall

include engagement with labor unions, community organizations, and industries, and place a special emphasis on communities hit hardest by the pandemic.

Sec. 3. Protecting Other Categories of Workers from COVID-19. (a) The Secretary of Labor, acting through the Assistant Secretary of Labor for Occupational Safety and Health and consistent with applicable law, shall:

(i) coordinate with States that have occupational safety and health plans approved under section 18 of the Occupational Safety and Health Act (Act) (29 U.S.C. 667) to seek to ensure that workers covered by such plans are adequately protected from COVID-19, consistent with any revised guidance or emergency temporary standards issued by OSHA; and

(ii) in States that do not have such plans, consult with State and local government entities with responsibility for public employee safety and health and with public employee unions to bolster protection from COVID-19 for public sector workers.

(b) The Secretary of Agriculture, the Secretary of Labor, the Secretary of Health and Human Services, the Secretary of Transportation, and the Secretary of Energy, in consultation with the heads of any other appropriate agencies, shall, consistent with applicable law, explore mechanisms to protect workers not protected under the Act so that they remain healthy and safe on the job during the COVID-19 pandemic.

(c) The Secretary of Labor, acting through the Assistant Secretary of Labor for Mine Safety and Health, shall consider whether any emergency temporary standards on COVID-19 applicable to coal and metal or non-metal mines are necessary, and if such standards are determined to be necessary and consistent with applicable law, issue them as soon as practicable.

Sec. 4. General Provisions. (a) Nothing in this order shall be construed to impair or otherwise affect:

(i) the authority granted by law to an executive department or agency, or the head thereof; or

(ii) the functions of the Director of the Office of Management and Budget relating to budgetary, administrative, or legislative proposals.

(b) This order shall be implemented consistent with applicable law and subject to the availability of appropriations.

(c) This order is not intended to, and does not, create any right or benefit, substantive or procedural, enforceable at law or in equity by any party against the United States, its departments, agencies, or entities, its officers, employees, or agents, or any other person.

EXECUTIVE ORDER

PROMOTING COVID-19 SAFETY IN DOMESTIC AND INTERNATIONAL TRAVEL

By the authority vested in me as President by the Constitution and the

laws of the United States of America, it is hereby ordered as follows:

Section 1. Policy. Science-based public health measures are critical to

preventing the spread of coronavirus disease 2019 (COVID-19) by travelers

within the United States and those who enter the country from abroad. The

Centers for Disease Control and Prevention (CDC), the Surgeon General, and

the National Institutes of Health have concluded that mask-wearing, physical

distancing, appropriate ventilation, and timely testing can mitigate the risk

of travelers spreading COVID-19. Accordingly, to save lives and allow all

Americans, including the millions of people employed in the transportation

industry, to travel and work safely, it is the policy of my Administration to

implement these public health measures consistent with CDC guidelines on

public modes of transportation and at ports of entry to the United States.

Sec. 2. Immediate Action to Require Mask-Wearing on

Certain Domestic Modes of Transportation.

(a) Mask Requirement. The Secretary of Labor, the Secretary of Health and Human Services (HHS), the Secretary of Transportation (including through the Administrator of the Federal Aviation Administration (FAA)), the Secretary of Homeland Security (including through the Administrator of the Transportation Security Administration (TSA) and the Commandant of the United States Coast Guard), and the heads of any other executive departments and agencies (agencies) that have relevant regulatory authority (heads of agencies) shall immediately take action, to the extent appropriate and consistent with applicable law, to require masks to be worn in compliance with CDC guidelines in or on:

(i)   airports;

(ii) commercial aircraft;

(iii) trains;

(iv) public maritime vessels, including ferries;

(v)   intercity bus services; and

(vi) all forms of public transportation as defined in section 5302 of title 49, United States Code.

(b) Consultation. In implementing this section, the heads of agencies shall consult, as appropriate, with interested parties, including State, local, Tribal, and territorial officials; industry and union representatives from the transportation sector; and consumer representatives.

(c) Exceptions. The heads of agencies may make categorical or case-by-case exceptions to policies developed under this section, consistent with applicable law, to the extent that doing so is necessary or required by law. If the heads of agencies do make exceptions, they shall require alternative and appropriate safeguards, and shall document all exceptions in writing.

(d) Preemption. To the extent permitted by applicable law, the heads of agencies shall ensure that any action taken to implement this section does not preempt State, local, Tribal, and territorial laws or rules imposing public health measures that are more protective of public health than those required by the heads of agencies.

(e) Coordination. The Coordinator of the COVID-19 Response and Counselor to the President (COVID-19 Response Coordinator) shall coordinate the implementation of this section. The heads of agencies shall update the COVID-19 Response Coordinator on their progress in implementing this section, including any categorical exceptions established under subsection (c) of this section, within 7 days of the date of this order and regularly thereafter. The heads of agencies are encouraged to bring to the attention of the COVID-19 Response Coordinator any questions regarding the scope or implementation of this section.

Sec. 3. Action to Implement Additional Public

Health Measures for Domestic Travel.

(a) Recommendations. The Secretary of Transportation (including through the Administrator of the FAA) and the Secretary of Homeland Security (including through the Administrator of the TSA and the Commandant of the Coast Guard), in consultation with the Director of CDC, shall promptly provide to the COVID-19 Response Coordinator recommendations concerning how their respective agencies may impose additional public health measures for domestic travel.

(b) Consultation. In implementing this section, the Secretary of Transportation and the Secretary of Homeland Security shall engage with interested parties, including State, local, Tribal, and territorial officials; industry and union representatives from the transportation sector; and consumer representatives.

Sec. 4. Support for State, Local, Tribal, and Territorial Authorities. The COVID-19 Response Coordinator, in coordination with the Secretary of Transportation and the heads of any other relevant agencies, shall promptly identify and inform agencies of options to incentivize, support, and encourage widespread mask-wearing and physical distancing on public modes of transportation, consistent with CDC guidelines and applicable law.

Sec. 5. International Travel.

(a) Policy. It is the policy of my Administration that, to the extent feasible, travelers seeking to enter the United States from a foreign country shall be:

(i) required to produce proof of a recent negative COVID-19 test prior to entry; and

(ii) required to comply with other applicable CDC guidelines

concerning international travel, including recommended periods of self-

quarantine or self-isolation after entry into the United States.

(b) Air Travel.

(i) The Secretary of HHS, including through the Director of CDC, and

in coordination with the Secretary of Transportation (including through

the Administrator of the FAA) and the Secretary of Homeland Security

(including through the Administrator of the TSA), shall, within 14 days of

the date of this order, assess the CDC order of January 12, 2021, regarding

the requirement of a negative COVID-19 test result for airline passengers

traveling into the United States, in light of subsection (a) of this section.

Based on such assessment, the Secretary of HHS and the Secretary of

Homeland Security shall take any further appropriate regulatory action, to

the extent feasible and consistent with CDC guidelines and applicable law.

Such assessment and regulatory action shall include consideration of:

(A) the timing and types of COVID-19 tests that should satisfy

the negative test requirement, including consideration of

additional testing immediately prior to departure;

(B) the proof of test results that travelers should be required to provide;

(C) the feasibility of implementing alternative and sufficiently protective

public health measures, such as testing, self-quarantine, and self-

isolation on arrival, for travelers entering the United States from

countries where COVID-19 tests are inaccessible, particularly where such

inaccessibility of tests would affect the ability of United States citizens

and lawful permanent residents to return to the United States; and

(D) measures to prevent fraud.

(ii) The Secretary of HHS, in coordination with the Secretary of Transportation

(including through the Administrator of the FAA) and the Secretary of Homeland

Security (including through the Administrator of the TSA), shall promptly provide

to the President, through the COVID-19 Response Coordinator, a plan for how the

Secretary and other Federal Government actors could implement the policy stated

in subsection (a) of this section with respect to CDC-recommended periods of self-

quarantine or self-isolation after a flight to the United States from a foreign country,

as he deems appropriate and consistent with applicable law. The plan shall identify

agencies' tools and mechanisms to assist travelers in complying with such policy.

(iii) The Secretary of State, in consultation with the Secretary of HHS (including

through the Director of CDC), the Secretary of Transportation (including

through the Administrator of the FAA), and the Secretary of Homeland Security,

shall seek to consult with foreign governments, the World Health Organization, the International Civil Aviation Organization, the International Air Transport Association, and any other relevant stakeholders to establish guidelines for public health measures associated with safe international travel, including on aircraft and at ports of entry. Any such guidelines should address quarantine, testing, COVID-19 vaccination, follow-up testing and symptom-monitoring, air filtration requirements, environmental decontamination standards, and contact tracing.

(c) Land Travel. The Secretary of State, in consultation with the Secretary of HHS, the Secretary of Transportation, the Secretary of Homeland Security, and the Director of CDC, shall immediately commence diplomatic outreach to the governments of Canada and Mexico regarding public health protocols for land ports of entry. Based on this diplomatic engagement, within 14 days of the date of this order, the Secretary of HHS (including through the Director of CDC), the Secretary of Transportation, and the Secretary of Homeland Security shall submit to the President a plan to implement appropriate public health measures at land ports of entry. The plan should implement CDC guidelines, consistent with applicable law, and take into account the operational considerations relevant to the different populations who enter the United States by land.

(d) Sea Travel. The Secretary of Homeland Security, through the Commandant of the Coast Guard and in consultation with the Secretary of HHS and the Director of CDC, shall, within 14 days of the date of this order, submit to the President a plan to implement appropriate public health measures at sea ports. The plan should implement CDC guidelines, consistent with applicable law, and take into account operational considerations.

(e) International Certificates of Vaccination or Prophylaxis. Consistent with applicable law, the Secretary of State, the Secretary of HHS, and the Secretary of Homeland Security (including through the Administrator of the TSA), in coordination with any relevant international organizations, shall assess the feasibility of linking COVID-19 vaccination to International Certificates of Vaccination or Prophylaxis (ICVP) and producing electronic versions of ICVPs.

(f) Coordination. The COVID-19 Response Coordinator, in consultation with the Assistant to the President for National Security Affairs and the Assistant to the President for Domestic Policy, shall coordinate the implementation of this section. The Secretary of State, the Secretary of HHS, the Secretary of Transportation, and the Secretary of Homeland Security shall update the COVID-19 Response Coordinator on their progress in implementing this section within 7 days of the date of this order and regularly thereafter. The heads of all agencies are encouraged to bring to the attention of the COVID-19 Response Coordinator any questions regarding the scope or implementation of this section.

Sec. 6. General Provisions. (a) Nothing in this order shall be construed to impair or otherwise affect:

(i) the authority granted by law to an executive

department or agency, or the head thereof; or

(ii) the functions of the Director of the Office of Management and Budget

relating to budgetary, administrative, or legislative proposals.

(b) This order shall be implemented consistent with applicable

law and subject to the availability of appropriations.

(c) This order is not intended to, and does not, create any right

or benefit, substantive or procedural, enforceable at law or in equity

by any party against the United States, its departments, agencies, or

entities, its officers, employees, or agents, or any other person.

THE WHITE HOUSE,

EXECUTIVE ORDER

ENSURING AN EQUITABLE PANDEMIC RESPONSE AND RECOVERY

By the authority vested in me as President by the Constitution and the laws of the United States of America, and in order to address the disproportionate and severe impact of coronavirus disease 2019 (COVID-19) on communities of color and other underserved populations, it is hereby ordered as follows:

Section 1. Purpose. The COVID-19 pandemic has exposed and exacerbated severe and pervasive health and social inequities in America. For instance, people of color experience systemic and structural racism in many facets of our society and are more likely to become sick and die from COVID-19. The lack of complete data, disaggregated by race and ethnicity, on COVID-19 infection, hospitalization, and mortality rates, as well as underlying health and social vulnerabilities, has further hampered efforts to ensure an equitable pandemic response. Other communities, often obscured in the data, are also disproportionately affected by COVID-19, including sexual and gender minority groups, those living with disabilities, and those living at the margins of our economy. Observed inequities in rural and Tribal communities, territories, and other geographically isolated communities require

a place-based approach to data collection and the response. Despite increased

State and local efforts to address these inequities, COVID-19's disparate impact on

communities of color and other underserved populations remains unrelenting.

Addressing this devastating toll is both a moral imperative and

pragmatic policy. It is impossible to change the course of the pandemic

without tackling it in the hardest-hit communities. In order to identify and

eliminate health and social inequities resulting in disproportionately higher

rates of exposure, illness, and death, I am directing a Government-wide

effort to address health equity. The Federal Government must take swift

action to prevent and remedy differences in COVID-19 care and outcomes

within communities of color and other underserved populations.

Sec. 2. COVID-19 Health Equity Task Force. There is

established within the Department of Health and Human Services

(HHS) a COVID-19 Health Equity Task Force (Task Force).

(a) Membership. The Task Force shall consist of the Secretary of HHS; an

individual designated by the Secretary of HHS to Chair the Task Force (COVID-19

Health Equity Task Force Chair); the heads of such other executive departments,

agencies, or offices (agencies) as the Chair may invite; and up to 20 members

from sectors outside of the Federal Government appointed by the President.

(i) Federal members may designate, to perform the Task Force functions of the member, a senior-level official who is a part of the member's agency and a full-time officer or employee of the Federal Government.

(ii) Nonfederal members shall include individuals with expertise and lived experience relevant to groups suffering disproportionate rates of illness and death in the United States; individuals with expertise and lived experience relevant to equity in public health, health care, education, housing, and community-based services; and any other individuals with expertise the President deems relevant. Appointments shall be made without regard to political affiliation and shall reflect a diverse set of perspectives.

(iii) Members of the Task Force shall serve without compensation for their work on the Task Force, but members shall be allowed travel expenses, including per diem in lieu of subsistence, as authorized by law for persons serving intermittently in the Government service (5 U.S.C. 5701-5707).

(iv) At the direction of the Chair, the Task Force may establish subgroups consisting exclusively of Task Force members or their designees under this section, as appropriate.

(b) Mission and Work.

(i) Consistent with applicable law and as soon as practicable, the Task Force shall provide specific recommendations to the President, through the Coordinator of the COVID-19 Response and Counselor to the President (COVID-19 Response Coordinator), for mitigating the health inequities caused or exacerbated by the COVID-19 pandemic and for preventing such inequities in the future. The recommendations shall include:

(A) recommendations for how agencies and State, local, Tribal, and territorial officials can best allocate COVID-19 resources, in light of disproportionately high rates of COVID-19 infection, hospitalization, and mortality in certain communities and disparities in COVID-19 outcomes by race, ethnicity, and other factors, to the extent permitted by law;

(B) recommendations for agencies with responsibility for disbursing COVID-19 relief funding regarding how to disburse funds in a manner that advances equity; and

(C) recommendations for agencies regarding effective, culturally aligned communication, messaging, and outreach to communities of color and other underserved populations.

(ii) The Task Force shall submit a final report to the COVID-19 Response Coordinator addressing any ongoing health inequities faced by COVID-19 survivors that may merit a public health response, describing the factors that contributed to disparities in COVID-19 outcomes, and recommending actions to combat such disparities in future pandemic responses.

(c) Data Collection. To address the data shortfalls identified in section

1 of this order, and consistent with applicable law, the Task Force shall:

(i) collaborate with the heads of relevant agencies, consistent with the

Executive Order entitled "Ensuring a Data-Driven Response to COVID-19

and Future High-Consequence Public Health Threats," to develop

recommendations for expediting data collection for communities of

color and other underserved populations and identifying data sources,

proxies, or indices that would enable development of short-term targets

for pandemic-related actions for such communities and populations;

(ii) develop, in collaboration with the heads of relevant agencies, a set of longer-

term recommendations to address these data shortfalls and other foundational

data challenges, including those relating to data intersectionality, that must

be tackled in order to better prepare and respond to future pandemics; and

(iii) submit the recommendations described in this subsection to

the President, through the COVID-19 Response Coordinator.

(d) External Engagement. Consistent with the objectives set out

in this order and with applicable law, the Task Force may seek the views

of health professionals; policy experts; State, local, Tribal, and territorial

health officials; faith-based leaders; businesses; health providers; community

organizations; those with lived experience with homelessness, incarceration, discrimination, and other relevant issues; and other stakeholders.

(e) Administration. Insofar as the Federal Advisory Committee Act, as amended (5 U.S.C. App.), may apply to the Task Force, any functions of the President under the Act, except for those in section 6 of the Act, shall be performed by the Secretary of HHS in accordance with the guidelines that have been issued by the Administrator of General Services. HHS shall provide funding and administrative support for the Task Force to the extent permitted by law and within existing appropriations. The Chair shall convene regular meetings of the Task Force, determine its agenda, and direct its work. The Chair shall designate an Executive Director of the Task Force, who shall coordinate the work of the Task Force and head any staff assigned to the Task Force.

(f) Termination. Unless extended by the President, the Task Force shall terminate within 30 days of accomplishing the objectives set forth in this order, including the delivery of the report and recommendations specified in this section, or 2 years from the date of this order, whichever comes first.

Sec. 3. Ensuring an Equitable Pandemic Response. To address the inequities identified in section 1 of this order, it is hereby directed that:

(a) The Secretary of Agriculture, the Secretary of Labor, the Secretary of HHS, the Secretary of Housing and Urban Development, the Secretary of Education, the Administrator of the Environmental Protection Agency, and the heads of all other agencies with authorities or responsibilities relating to the pandemic response and recovery shall, as appropriate and consistent with applicable law:

(i) consult with the Task Force to strengthen equity data collection, reporting, and use related to COVID-19;

(ii) assess pandemic response plans and policies to determine whether personal protective equipment, tests, vaccines, therapeutics, and other resources have been or will be allocated equitably, including by considering:

(A) the disproportionately high rates of COVID-19 infection, hospitalization, and mortality in certain communities; and

(B) any barriers that have restricted access to preventive measures, treatment, and other health services for high-risk populations;

(iii) based on the assessments described in subsection (a)(ii) of this section, modify pandemic response plans and policies to advance equity, with consideration to:

(A) the effect of proposed policy changes on the distribution of resources to, and access to health care by, communities of color and other underserved populations;

(B) the effect of proposed policy changes on agencies' ability to collect, analyze, and report data necessary to monitor and evaluate the impact of pandemic response plans and policies on communities of color and other underserved populations; and

(C) policy priorities expressed by communities that have suffered disproportionate rates of illness and death as a result of the pandemic;

(iv) strengthen enforcement of anti-discrimination requirements pertaining

to the availability of, and access to, COVID-19 care and treatment; and

(v) partner with States, localities, Tribes, and territories to explore

mechanisms to provide greater assistance to individuals and families

experiencing disproportionate economic or health effects from COVID-19,

such as by expanding access to food, housing, child care, or income support.

(b) The Secretary of HHS shall:

(i) provide recommendations to State, local, Tribal, and territorial leaders

on how to facilitate the placement of contact tracers and other workers

in communities that have been hardest hit by the pandemic, recruit such

workers from those communities, and connect such workers to existing health

workforce training programs and other career advancement programs; and

(ii) conduct an outreach campaign to promote vaccine trust and uptake

among communities of color and other underserved populations with

higher levels of vaccine mistrust due to discriminatory medical treatment

and research, and engage with leaders within those communities.

Sec. 4. General Provisions. (a) Nothing in this order

shall be construed to impair or otherwise affect:

(i) the authority granted by law to an executive

department or agency, or the head thereof; or

(ii) the functions of the Director of the Office of Management and Budget

relating to budgetary, administrative, or legislative proposals.

(b) This order shall be implemented consistent with

applicable law and subject to the availability of appropriations.

(c) This order is not intended to, and does not, create any right

or benefit, substantive or procedural, enforceable at law or in equity

by any party against the United States, its departments, agencies, or

entities, its officers, employees, or agents, or any other person.

THE WHITE HOUSE,

NATIONAL SECURITY DIRECTIVE

SUBJECT: United States Global Leadership to Strengthen
the International COVID-19 Response and to
Advance Global Health Security and Biological
Preparedness

The coronavirus disease 2019 (COVID-19) pandemic is a grave reminder that biological threats, whether naturally occurring, accidental, or deliberate, can have significant and potentially existential consequences for humanity. This directive reaffirms Executive Order 13747 of November 4, 2016, which made clear that these threats pose global challenges that require global solutions. United States international engagement to combat COVID-19 and advance global health security and biopreparedness is thus an urgent priority -- to save lives, promote economic recovery, and develop resilience against future biological catastrophes. My Administration will treat epidemic and pandemic preparedness, health security, and global health as top national security priorities, and will work with other nations to combat COVID-19 and seek to create a world that is safe and secure from biological threats.

Section 1. Strengthening and Reforming the World Health Organization. On January 20, 2021, the United States reversed its decision to withdraw from the World Health Organization (WHO) by submitting a letter to the United Nations Secretary-General informing him of the President's decision that the United States will remain a member of the organization. Accordingly, the Assistant to the President for National Security Affairs (APNSA) shall, in coordination with the Secretary of State, the Secretary of Health and Human Services (HHS), the heads of other relevant executive departments and agencies (agencies), and the Coordinator of the COVID-19 Response and Counselor to the President (COVID-19 Response Coordinator), provide to the President within 30 days of the date of this directive recommendations on how the United States can: (1) exercise leadership at the WHO and work with partners to lead and reinvigorate the international COVID-19 response; (2) participate in international efforts to advance global health, health security, and the prevention of future biological catastrophes; and (3) otherwise strengthen and reform the WHO.

Sec. 2. United States Leadership in the Global Response to COVID-19.

(a) COVID-19 Global Vaccination, Research, and Development. In order to support global vaccination and research and development for treatments, tests, and vaccines:

(i) The Secretary of State and the Secretary of HHS shall inform the WHO and Gavi, the Vaccine Alliance, of the United States' intent to support the Access to COVID-19 Tools (ACT) Accelerator and join the multilateral vaccine distribution facility, known as the COVID-19 Vaccine Global Access (COVAX) Facility. The Secretaries shall also promptly deliver to the President, through the APNSA and the COVID-19 Response Coordinator, a framework for donating surplus vaccines, once there is sufficient supply in the United States, to countries in need, including through the COVAX Facility.

(ii) The Secretary of State and the Secretary of HHS, in coordination with the heads of other relevant agencies, shall promptly deliver to the APNSA and the COVID-19 Response Coordinator a plan for engaging with and strengthening multilateral initiatives focused on the global COVID-19 response, including the organizations identified in section 2(a)(i) and other initiatives focused on equitable development and distribution of vaccines, therapeutics, tests, and personal protective equipment, such as the Coalition for Epidemic Preparedness Innovations and the Global Fund to Fight AIDS, Tuberculosis and Malaria.

(b) Health, Diplomatic, and Humanitarian Response to COVID-19. In order to enable the United States to play an active role in the international COVID-19 public health and humanitarian response, including with respect to the pandemic's secondary effects:

(i) The Secretary of State, in coordination with the Secretary of HHS, the Administrator of the UnitedStates Agency for International Development (USAID), the Director of the Centers for Disease Control and Prevention (CDC), and the heads of other relevant agencies, shall promptly develop and submit to the President, through the APNSA and the COVID-19 Response Coordinator, a Government-wide plan to combat the global COVID-19 pandemic, which shall identify principal strategic objectives, corresponding lines of effort, and lead agencies.

(ii)   The Secretary of State shall, in coordination with the heads of other relevant agencies, promptly review and, as necessary, adjust the United States' current and planned future deployments of public health, health security, and health diplomacy personnel overseas focused on the COVID-19 response, taking into account best practices for such deployments from partner nations' COVID-19 response strategies.

(iii) Within 14 days of the date of this directive or as soon as possible thereafter, the Secretary of State shall develop, in consultation with the Secretary of HHS, the Representative of the United States to the United Nations, the Administrator of USAID, and the Director of the CDC, a diplomatic outreach plan for enhancing the United States' response to the COVID-19 pandemic, with a focus on engaging partner nations, the United Nations (including the United Nations Security Council), and other multilateral stakeholders on:

(A) the financing of and capacity for strengthening the global COVID-19 response;

(B) the provision of assistance, including in humanitarian settings and to mitigate secondary impacts of the COVID-19 pandemic such as food insecurity and gender-based violence; and

(C) the provision of support, including with the United Nations and other relevant multilateral fora, for the capacity of the most vulnerable communities to prevent, detect, respond to, mitigate, and recover from impacts of COVID-19.

(c) COVID-19 Sanctions Relief. The Secretary of State, the Secretary of the Treasury, and the Secretary of Commerce, in consultation with the Secretary of HHS and the Administrator of USAID, shall promptly review existing United States and multilateral financial and economic sanctions to evaluate whether they are unduly hindering responses to the COVID-19 pandemic, and provide recommendations to the President, through the APNSA and the COVID-19 Response Coordinator, for any changes in approach.

Sec. 3. Review of Funding for COVID-19 Response and Global Health Security and Biodefense. In order to ensure that global health security considerations are central to United States foreign policy, global health policy, and national security, the Director of the Office of Management and Budget shall, in coordination with the heads of relevant agencies and the APNSA:

(a) review the funding allocated for the COVID-19 response, including the secondary impacts of the pandemic, as well as for global health security, global health, pandemic preparedness, and biodefense; and

(b) provide the President with an assessment of whether that funding, as well as funding for subsequent budgetary years, is sufficient to support operations and administrative needs related to the COVID-19 response, as well as future global health security, global health, pandemic preparedness, and biodefense needs.

Sec. 4. Financing for Global Health Security. In order to develop a health security financing mechanism, make strategic use of multilateral and bilateral channels and institutions, and assist developing countries in preparing for, preventing, detecting, and responding to COVID-19 and other infectious disease threats:

(a) The APNSA, in coordination with the Secretary of State, the Secretary of the Treasury, the Secretary of HHS, the Administrator of USAID, the Chief Executive Officer of the United States International Development Finance Corporation, and the heads of other agencies providing foreign assistance and development financing, shall promptly provide to the President recommendations for creating an enduring international catalytic financing mechanism for advancing and improving existing bilateral and multilateral approaches to global health security.

(b) The Secretary of the Treasury shall promptly provide to the President, through the APNSA, a strategy on how the United States can promote in international financial institutions, including the World Bank Group and International Monetary Fund, financing, relief, and other policies that are aligned with and support the goals of combating COVID-19 and strengthening global health security.

Sec. 5. Advancing Global Health Security and Epidemic and Pandemic Preparedness.

(a) The APNSA shall:

(i) coordinate the Federal Government's efforts to prepare for, prevent, detect, respond to, and recover from biological events, and to advance global health security, international pandemic preparedness, and global health resilience;

(ii) coordinate the development of priorities for, and elevate United States leadership and assistance in support of, the Global Health Security Agenda;

(iii) conduct, in coordination with the heads of relevant agencies, a review of existing United States health security policies and strategies and develop recommendations for how the Federal Government may update them, including by, as appropriate: developing stronger global institutions focused on harmonizing crisis response for emerging biological events and public health emergencies; taking steps to strengthen the global pandemic supply chain and address any barriers to the timely delivery of supplies in response to a pandemic; working with partner countries and international organizations to strengthen and implement the International Health Regulations; reducing racial and ethnic disparities in the COVID-19 global response and disproportionate impacts on marginalized and indigenous communities, women and girls, and other groups; reviewing and developing priorities for multilateral fora aimed at reducing the risk of deliberate or accidental biological events; combating antimicrobial resistance; and fighting climate change as a driver of health threats; and

(iv) develop, in coordination with the Secretary of State, the Secretary of HHS, the Administrator of USAID, the Director of the CDC, and the heads of other relevant agencies, protocols for coordinating and deploying a global response to emerging high-consequence infectious disease threats. These protocols should outline the respective roles for relevant agencies in facilitating and supporting such response operations, including by establishing standard operating procedures for how USAID and the CDC coordinate their response efforts.

(b) The APNSA, in coordination with the COVID-19 Response Coordinator, the Assistant to the President for Domestic Policy, and the heads of relevant agencies, shall promptly develop a plan for establishing an interagency National Center for Epidemic Forecasting and Outbreak Analytics and modernizing global early warning and trigger systems for scaling action to prevent, detect, respond to, and recover from emerging biological threats.

(c) The Secretary of State and the Representative of the United States to the United Nations shall provide to the President, through the APNSA, recommendations regarding steps the United States should take to encourage or support the establishment of a new position in the office of the United Nations Secretary-General of a facilitator for high-consequence biological threats, particularly for events involving significant collaboration and equities across the United Nations.

(d) To assist in the Federal Government's efforts to provide warning of pandemics, protect our biotechnology infrastructure from cyber attacks and intellectual property theft, identify and monitor biological threats from states and non-state actors, provide validation of foreign data and response efforts, and assess strategic challenges and opportunities from emerging biotechnologies, the Director of National Intelligence shall:

(i) Review the collection and reporting capabilities in the United States Intelligence Community (IC) related to pandemics and the full range of high-consequence biological threats and develop a plan for how the IC may strengthen and prioritize such capabilities, including through organizational changes or the creation of National Intelligence Manager and National Intelligence Officer positions focused on biological threats, global public health, and biotechnology;

(ii) Develop and submit to the President, through the APNSA and the COVID-19 Response Coordinator, a National Intelligence Estimate on (A) the impact of COVID-19 on national and economic security; and (B) current, emerging, reemerging, potential, and future biological risks to national and economic security; and

(iii) In coordination with the Secretary of State, the Secretary of Defense, the Secretary of HHS, the Director of the CDC, the Administrator of USAID, the Director of the Office of Science and Technology Policy, and the heads of other relevant agencies, promptly develop and submit to the APNSA an analysis of the security implications of biological threats that can be incorporated into modeling, simulation, course of action analysis, and other analyses.

Sec. 6. General Provisions. (a) Nothing in this directive shall be construed to impair or otherwise affect:

(i) the authority granted by law to an executive department or agency, or the head thereof; or

(ii) the functions of the Director of the Office of Management and Budget relating to budgetary, administrative, or legislative proposals.

(b) This directive shall be implemented consistent with applicable law and subject to the availability of appropriations.

(c) This directive is not intended to, and does not, create any right or benefit, substantive or procedural, enforceable at law or in equity by any party against the United States, its departments, agencies, or entities, its officers, employees, or agents, or any other person.

NOTES

NOTES

NOTES

NOTES

NOTES

NOTES

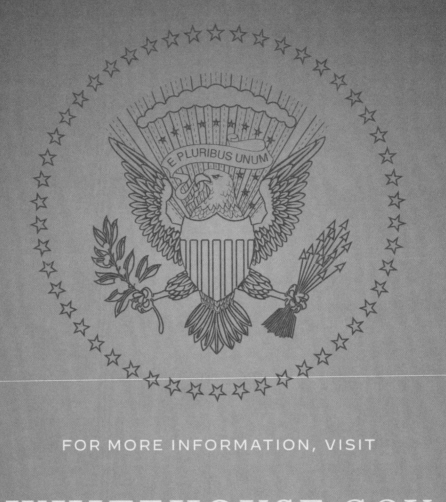

FOR MORE INFORMATION, VISIT

WHITEHOUSE.GOV

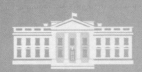